Abortion and the
Unwanted Child

Abortion
and
the
Unwanted Child

The California Committee
on Therapeutic Abortion

edited by Carl Reiterman

Springer Publishing Company, Inc., New York City

The Authors

Mildred B. Beck

M.S.W., Former Chief, Research Support Section, Center for Epidemiologic Studies, National Institute of Mental Health, and currently Acting Chief, Office of Information, National Center for Family Planning Services, Health Services and Mental Health Administration, U.S. Department of Health, Education, and Welfare, Rockville, Maryland

Garrett Hardin

Ph.D., Professor of Biology, University of California, Santa Barbara

Jimmye Kimmey

Executive Director, Association for the Study of Abortion, New York City

E. James Lieberman

M.D., Former Chief, Center for Studies of Child and Family Mental Health, National Institute of Mental Health, Bethesda, Maryland; Assistant Clinical Professor of Psychiatry, Howard University School of Medicine, Washington, D.C., Visiting Lecturer on Maternal and Child Health, Harvard School of Public Health

Charlotte F. Muller

Ph.D., Professor, Center for Social Research, City University of New York

Maurine Neuberger

Former United States Senator from Oregon and Chairman, 1968 Citizens' Advisory Council on the Status of Women

v

Edmund W. Overstreet

M.D., Professor and Vice-Chairman, Department of Obstetrics and Gynecology, University of California Medical Center, San Francisco

Sally Provence

M.D., Professor of Pediatrics, Yale University Child Study Center, New Haven, Connecticut

Carl Reiterman

Ph.D., Assistant Professor of Sociology, University of San Francisco, Lecturer in Public Health Demography, School of Public Health, University of California, Berkeley, and Lecturer in Epidemiology, School of Medicine, University of California, San Francisco

Ruth Roemer

J.D., Associate Researcher in Health Law, Institute of Government and Public Affairs, University of California, Los Angeles

Norma G. Zarky

LL.B., Member, Board of Governors, Beverly Hills Bar Association and Member, Board of Trustees, Exceptional Children's Foundation

Preface

If beleaguered man is to survive on his infinitesimal planet, achieving through a birth- rather than a death-rate solution the population balance necessitated by his round earth's four corners, the birth of unwanted children must be substantially eliminated. Further, the term "unwanted" must include not only unwanted children produced by excessively fertile parents, but the excess of births over deaths which is the sole factor responsible for continued population increase at the planetary level.

In this effort, abortion will almost certainly continue to play a major part.

This book is based on papers delivered at the California Conference on Abortion, held in San Francisco on 9-11 May 1969. Four papers have been added: one dealing with recent legislative and judicial developments; another focused on the question of payment for medical care in abortion cases; a survey of the fate of more than a hundred children who were born after their mothers had been refused a therapeutic abortion; and a brief essay of my own. Also, because of its interest and importance, the opinion of the California Supreme Court in *People v. Belous* is included. We believe that all of these papers will contribute to the ongoing discussion of this vital problem.

I am grateful to Professor Garrett Hardin, the chairman of the conference, for his invitation to serve as editor of this book, and for much sound advice during the editing process. I also thank the organizing committee, the sponsors, the participants, and especially those who contributed the papers on which the book is based. "One Hundred and Twenty Children Born after Application for Therapeutic Abortion Refused" is reprinted with the kind permission of the authors, Hans Forssman, M.D., and Inga Thuwe. Finally, I thank the National Institute of Mental Health for the grant (U.S. Public Health Service grant L R13 MH18017-01) which greatly facilitated this project.

Berkeley   Carl Reiterman
November 1970

vii

*The law in its majestic equality forbids
the rich as well as the poor to sleep under
bridges, to beg in the streets, and to steal bread.*

Anatole France

Contents

ix

Chapter 1

We Need Abortion for the Children's Sake

Garrett Hardin

Many changes concerning abortion have taken place in the past three years, not so much in the law as in the climate of opinion. The law has been changed in California as well as in a number of other states. Senator Anthony Beilenson candidly refers to the law that he pushed through the California legislature as "my crummy little law"—he knew it was not the best of all laws, but he felt it was the best law that he could get through the legislature at that time. Until a better law can be passed, we have to live with this one. How we can best live with it, and what we might do about improving it, are major concerns here.

Looking back over the past few years I am astonished to see how our ideas have changed. In 1966 any meeting on abortion necessarily had to spend a considerable amount of time discussing the religious angle. Now we ignore it most of the time. Carl Reiterman, carrying out a very thorough analysis of Catholic literature, has shown that it is a mistake to see the controversy over contraception merely as a battle waged between Catholics and non-Catholics. For the past generation, the battle among Catholics themselves on this issue has been far fiercer(1).

Those of us who lecture in public on abortion realize that the history of contraception is being repeated with abortion, which is by definition a method of birth control(2). Many Catholic women have buttonholed me to tell me about their abortions. They're not ashamed of them. They know they have resorted to this form of birth control out of consideration for their families. It is principally Catholic men who are "hung up" on this issue. Unfortunately, men are the custodians of the dogma and sit in the halls of legislature.

Our greatest advance in the last decade has been in removing the taboo from the word "abortion." Five years ago many people thought it was courageous of me to discuss the subject in public. They were wrong, of course; but since this was a flattering error, I did not correct them. Now, no one flatters me in this way; everybody talks about abortion. Women candidly discuss their abortions in public meetings. Discovering that they are not alone, they gather strength to work for reform. And men, as they discover that "nice" women have abortions, sometimes have second thoughts about theological dogma and the laws.

Yet talking about the abortion problem is still not as easy as it should be. We still hear people say, "I'm not completely against abortion, but it seems to me a messy solution. Isn't contraception better? Why should we encourage women to be careless?"

Superficially, this seems a plausible stand to take, but implicit in it is an image of sex as only a matter of plumbing and pipes, of buttons and reflexes and cold-blooded "decisions." The reality is quite otherwise: richer, more complex—and sometimes more exasperating.

Why do women get pregnant? The easy way to "explain" things is with a name. Women get pregnant, we may be told, because they have a "maternal instinct." But when you inquire deeply it seems almost as though the reasons for getting pregnant are nearly as numerous as the number of pregnancies. One woman gets pregnant because she dislikes her husband and it gives her a ready excuse for avoiding intercourse. Another gets pregnant to punish her parents, or to make it difficult for her husband to accept a job transfer. Many women get pregnant because they don't know what else to do—that is, because perpetual motherhood is the only meaningful career they see open to them. As a matter of methodology we should refuse the "maternal instinct" explanation of pregnancy except as a last and most desperate resort. We know very little about the proximate causes of pregnancy. We need to know a great deal more if we are to eliminate unwanted pregnancies.

My inquiries into the reasons for pregnancy are confined almost entirely to college girls, so I do not hear the full range of reasons, nor am I exposed to a random sample. The most heartbreaking cases, those of impoverished mothers pregnant for the nth time, do not normally come my way. Even so, I have learned something.

When a college girl becomes pregnant one wonderingly asks, Why? Is it because she didn't know that intercourse had something to do with conception? Or didn't she know about contraception? Among the many cases that have come my way I have yet to find a girl who did not know the answer to both of these questions before she became pregnant.

Evidently, merely knowing in an intellectual way about the existence of pills, coils, foams, and diaphragms will not keep a girl from becoming pregnant. Some other sort of education is needed. But what kind?

Before we can begin to answer this question we need to have a deeper understanding of the reasons why a *technically* knowledgeable girl becomes pregnant when she does not wish to. There may be many reasons for this, but I will discuss only one very common reason, a reason that poses a serious problem to those responsible for sex education in the schools.

Why does a girl who knows about the pill get pregnant? *Because she wants to keep her virginity.* Over and over again I have found a common pattern of feeling and thinking responsible for unwanted pregnancies. The girl has been brought up to be a "good girl." Her parents have praised virginity, perhaps on moral grounds, perhaps on practical grounds. She has gotten the idea that it is good to remain a virgin until you are married, and bad (or at any rate, risky) not to. Losing one's virginity before marriage is, at the very least, bad manners.

As she moves out of the home environment and into an environment controlled by her peers she hears conflicting messages. These, reinforced by her hormones, suggest that there is something to be said for nonvirginity. She becomes ambivalent in her desires. She isn't quite sure what she wants to do, but one thing she is sure of: she could never be so cold-blooded as to ask a doctor to write her a prescription for contraceptive pills in advance of her first intercourse, or to fit her with a diaphragm. To do so would be "too calculating"; it would be to admit to herself that she had abandoned the ideal of virginity. She just couldn't do it. She doesn't *intend* to have intercourse.

But if she does have intercourse—and she just *might*—it will be because she has been "carried away" by passion, that things have gone beyond her control. That which is beyond her control is beyond good and evil. She is not responsible for what happens then. Thus, the "good girl" becomes pregnant precisely because of her virginal intentions. Without these virginal intentions it would be easy for her to make rational preparations for the coming loss of virginity. Even after the first intercourse the "good girl" continues to follow this perilous pattern for a while, for the same ambivalent reasons. Her boyfriend's psychological set may be not too different.

What is the answer to this problem? More "education"? And what kind of education?

Without taking sides, I think that there are two possible kinds of education that one could recommend, and they are diametrically opposed to each other. The first would include a greatly strengthened emphasis on the importance of virginity—on its moral value and also on its hygienic value (i.e., as the way to avoid contracting venereal disease). As an abstract proposition, one could argue that such an increased emphasis would increase the frequency of genuine virginity. But to be successful, of course, this kind of education would have to take place in a social setting in which all the meaningful authority figures in the girl's life were committed, without ambivalence, to the same ideal— and where are we to find such a setting these days?

The second kind of education would decrease the emphasis on virginity, not necessarily explicitly downgrading it, but perhaps merely ignoring it. Instead of emphasizing the desirability of virginity, we might emphasize the social sin of a girl's becoming pregnant without considering the interests of everyone else concerned. Victorian moralists would draw back at the thought of such an education; they would say that such an approach condones sexual intercourse among the unmarried. Perhaps they are right. Perhaps, to be successful, such an education would have to condone premarital intercourse, or even openly encourage it.

Whatever our personal tastes in sex education for the future, surely this much is clear: that we must more and more emphasize the *non-right* of the individual woman to continue a pregnancy in utter disregard of the interests of the significant persons in her life—her parents (if she is a dependent minor), her boyfriend, or her husband, and even society as a whole, since much of the cost of rearing and educating her child will be borne by society at large. Above all she must consider the interests of the child who will come into being if she allows the pregnancy to continue. If the total circumstances are such that the child born at a particular time and under particular circumstances will not receive a fair shake in life, then she should know—she should feel in her bones—that she has no right to continue the pregnancy.

Although what I've just said seems to imply that the pregnant woman is at fault for not having an abortion, this is seldom true. It is society that stands in the way, for though it approves of birth control in general, it disapproves of this particular form of birth control.

Most women who should have abortions want them for the best of all possible reasons: because they love children. For the sake of the children already born a woman wants desperately to avoid having one too many. For the sake of other children she may have several years later, she wants an abortion now. She knows that her time, her patience, and her love are not infinitely divisible. The final straw that breaks the camel's back does not break the legislator's back nor the theologian's. It breaks hers.

The Forssman and Thuwe Study, done in Sweden with meticulously selected controls, studied children born to mothers who had asked for abortions but had been refused. The children were 21 years old at the time of the study. The unwanted children were in poorer health than the wanted controls. They had a history of more psychiatric attention. They used alcohol more. The boys were, with greater frequency, rejected by the army. And the girls had babies earlier and married earlier, thus (no doubt) perpetuating their psychological problems into the next generation. For many of these troubles the taxpayers ultimately paid(3).

"But that was in Sweden. How do we know that it would be true in America?" We don't know. It would take at least 21 years to carry out a similar study in the United States. Since we lack long-term studies done in the United States, we must make do with such data as we have. We are not entirely without information. The "battered child" statistics are highly suggestive. It should alarm us all to learn that between 1963 and 1967, while infant mortality from all other causes fell, the rate of infant homicide rose by 28 percent. In this area, we can expect little good to come from the passage of more stringent laws against child battering. We must strike at the cause of the tragedies by doing away with all compulsory pregnancy, thus minimizing the frequency of unwanted births.

The realization that the welfare of children is the most important aspect of the abortion problem is important to stress when urging abortion legislation. Since legislators are called upon to vote funds for the care of children who are neglected in the home, they are acutely aware that what happens to children is a concern of society in general.

Before we can persuade legislators that access to medically competent abortion should be the acknowledged right of every woman, we would do well to convince them that the results of not acknowledging this right cost money. We need more studies to make the truth undeniable. I have no doubt that competently planned research will uncover a wealth of useful facts. In this field, as in so many others, economic interest and ethical interest fortunately coincide. Legislative acts that will diminish the taxes now being paid for the care of unwanted and unloved children will also diminish the amount of misery in the world.

For the future, I would urge that all abortion reformers give increasing attention to convincing those who are in power that it is to their interest to make women free. By this practical approach we can come closer to the day dreamed of by Margaret Sanger when she said: "The first right of every child is to be wanted, to be desired, to be planned with an intensity of love that gives it its title to being."

REFERENCES

1. Carl Reiterman. Birth Control and Catholics, *Journal for the Scientific Study of Religion 4*:2 (Spring, 1965):213-233.
2. The U.S. Department of Health, Education, and Welfare, for example, has defined birth control measures as "procedures deliberately employed to interfere at one or another stage with the normal sequence of events in the process of reproduction. They include methods to prevent the occurrence of conception (contraception) or to preclude the development of the conceptus (abortion)." *A Survey of Research on Reproduction Related to Birth and Population Control* (December 1962), p. 7. Ed.
3. Hans Forssman and Inga Thuwe. One Hundred and Twenty Children Born After Application for Therapeutic Abortion Refused. *Acta Psychiatrica Scandinavica 42* (1966):71-88. Appendix, pp. 123-145.

Chapter **2**

Abortion Law Reform in the United States

Jimmye Kimmey

The movement for abortion law reform in the United States is gaining momentum. There is increasing support from the public, as shown by public opinion polls and by the formation of state and local groups working for legislative change; there is increasing support for such change from national, state, and local religious, civic, and professional groups; and there is increasing activity on the legislative scene.

Specifically, in 1967 twenty-nine states considered abortion law reform legislation; in 1968 and 1969 more than thirty-five did so. Five states—California, Colorado, Georgia, North Carolina, and Maryland—had revised abortion laws in effect at the beginning of the 1969 term.

Three states—Arkansas, Kansas, and New Mexico enacted abortion reform bills introduced in 1969. These laws are based on the American Law Institute's Model Penal Code providing that "a licensed physician is justified in terminating a pregnancy if he believes there is substantial risk that continuance of the pregnancy would gravely impair the physical or mental health of the mother or that the child would be born with grave physical or mental defect, or that the pregnancy resulted from rape, incest or other felonious intercourse."

Out of a total of 49 abortion reform measures introduced in 1969, 29 were based on the American Law Institute's model, 12 provided only that abortions must be done by licensed physicians, four would have

Miss Kimmey's paper is presented in her individual capacity, not as a representative of The Association for the Study of Abortion, Inc.

7

repealed existing abortion statutes, and four were more restrictive than the ALI code.

This increasing legislative activity reflected increasing public acceptance of the essential justice of abortion reform. A survey by the National Opinion Research Center in 1965, together with the National Fertility Study of Westoff and Ryder, also in 1965, when compared with a Gallup Poll taken for the Population Council in late 1967, show an increasing proportion of respondents approving abortion for the same reasons. All three studies found substantial majorities favoring liberalizing the law along the lines of the ALI code. Furthermore, the minorities favoring abortion on request or for socio-economic reasons are substantial (one-quarter to one-third), and are growing.

Another index of the growth of support for abortion law reform is the increasing number of state and local groups working on this problem. In 1966, the Association for the Study of Abortion *Newsletter* listed six such groups, while the ASA *Newsletter* for Summer 1969 lists thirty-five state and local groups, plus two new national organizations.

The increasing support for more liberal abortion laws on the part of medical, regligious, and civic organizations is truly impressive. I will not try to provide a comprehensive list but will note some highlights: that the American Civil Liberties Union has called for freedom of choice in this matter is scarcely surprising, but few would have predicted that the American Baptist Convention would ask that abortion in the first twelve weeks of pregnancy be treated as an elective medical procedure. Who would have predicted that the Presbytery of New York City would ask for repeal of New York's abortion law? And, at least for some of us outside the area, the action of the Iowa Council of Churches in calling, in effect, for freedom of choice in this matter was a surprise.

Nor have the medical and health groups been silent. The American Public Health Association in 1968 stated its belief that "safe legal abortion should be available to all women" and called for the repeal of restrictive laws. The American Medical Association has lent its support to ALI-type reform, and the American College of Obstetricians and Gynecologists has gone even further, adopting this language from the liberal British law: "In determining whether or not there is . . . risk to health [sufficient to justify abortion], account may be taken of the patient's total environment, actual or reasonably foreseeable." Some state societies have been even more liberal, as for example, the Minnesota State Medical Association, which in 1968 adopted a committee report advocating a policy "designed to afford ethical physicians the right to exercise their sound medical judgment concerning therapeutic abortion just as they do in reaching any other medical decision."

Here, then, is a movement which evokes widespread interest and support from the general public, from professionals, and from politicians. The question is: What is the abortion law reform movement going to do with this growing support? Where is the movement going?

When, in the middle 60's, people in the abortion reform movement talked of abortion law reform, it seemed clear that the reform objective was to make it possible for a woman to have an abortion with no more difficulty than she now faces in arranging to have a baby. There were two feasible routes to that objective: legislative and judicial.

As for the legislative route, the political assessment in most states then was that, while repeal might be the quickest way to achieve the ultimate goal, it was impossible of immediate achievement and therefore it was felt that a good first step would be to settle for something like the American Law Institute's model code.

After a year or so the meaning of the word reform seemed to undergo a change. There were those in the movement who began to talk as if reform of abortion laws was an unworthy objective and as if the struggle to repeal those laws was the only fight worth waging. This development sent me to the dictionary where I found the following definition: "Reform . . . to amend or improve by change of form or removal of faults or abuses." It seems to me that any legislative development from an ALI-type bill to total repeal of any existing abortion law fits quite comfortably into this definition.

In any social movement there are those who refuse to compromise, who refuse to meet their opponents (or even their friends) half-way. The no-compromisers enjoy one great advantage—they can argue openly for their position on ideological grounds and therefore appear to themselves and others to be pure of heart. That sensation is, no doubt, a great source of energy, but it is apparently such a heady sensation that it sometimes induces blindness.

To what are the no-compromisers blindless? They are unable to see that, just as on occasion the good is the enemy of the excellent, so the perfect can be the enemy of the good. Fighting for the first-step ALI-type reform may either enhance or delay chances for the ultimate reform. What the no-compromisers fail to see is that this is not a question that can sensibly be argued in the abstract.

In political life it is necessary to choose one's tactics on the basis of political reality rather than on the basis of what one wishes political reality were like. Only when the actual political situation is understood can desired changes be initiated. It is not enough to be self-righteously right—it is necessary to be politically effective.

In some states, political realism leads to the conclusion that a bill limiting the practice of abortion to licensed physicians, or even one that calls for outright repeal of existing statutes, would have a real chance of passage. In such states, introduction of an ALI bill would be foolish. In other states, political reality dictates that getting even an ALI bill approved would be an achievement. In these states to insist on repeal or nothing would be foolish.

In 1969, the careful political assessment in some states was that a bill restricting abortions to licensed physicians had a real chance of passage, and in a few states the battle was very nearly won. In Kansas, for example, such a bill passed the Senate but the House added ALI-type provisions to the law as finally passed and signed. Thus, in some states, political reality seems on the verge of catching up with our hopes.

Through 1969 neither the political realists nor the no-compromisers were successful in getting the law repealed anywhere. And, what is worse, in some states the no-compromisers may have been detrimental to other reform efforts.

One branch of the no-compromisers—the radical feminists—may have been instrumental on occasion in defeating the move to reform the law short of their ideal. In New York and Minnesota, for example, such groups disrupted legislative hearings by shouting down even sympathetic testimony. There is no evidence that these groups have undertaken the less exciting but potentially more effective work of trying to influence legislators in less hostile ways.

Turning to the national scene, there are now two activist organizations which have differing approaches to the problem of abortion law reform. Whether these differing approaches will turn out to be in conflict remains to be seen.

The Abortion Reform Association, established in 1968, has as its objective lending assistance (including making grants) to state abortion reform groups around the country. ARA has made grants to groups that support ALI-type bills and to groups that support bills whose only restriction is that abortions be performed by licensed physicians. ARA's assumption is that an organization that is working for the passage of at least an ALI bill and that has done its political homework is worthy of support. Since ARA defines reform as covering the spectrum of change from ALI to outright repeal, it is clear that it will not oppose efforts at legislative change falling within those very broad limits. Its stated purpose is "to seek repeal of abortion laws where this seems to be politically feasible and to seek maximal liberalization of these laws where seeking repeal seems unrealistic."

The second new organization is the National Association for the Repeal of Abortion Laws which grew out of a conference held in Chicago in early 1969. While the name focuses on repeal, the organization also supports laws limiting the performance of abortion to licensed physicians.

The ultimate objective is to change medical practice. Thus it may be that disagreements over the content of legislation are not only debilitating to the movement but irrelevant to the goal. Since the vital constituency is the medical community, perhaps consideration should be given to the question of whether flamboyant tactics such as demonstrating, picketing hospitals, and disrupting legislative hearings will lose the respect of the medical community. If this respect is lost, changing the law may have only a limited impact on medical practice.

In fact, it may be that even if physicians are not offended, reform or repeal of the law would make less difference in medical practice than one might hope. We know, for example, that although voluntary sterilization is not illegal in any state patients often have a difficult time securing this medical service. Might this be in part because the physicians (and more especially the hospital administrator) feels no necessity to do something just because it is not illegal? If, under liberalized laws, physicians and hospitals still followed restrictive policies, it might turn out that the hope for changing medical practice would lie along the judicial route.

At present, the *Stewart v. Long Island College Hospital* case is on its way up the judicial ladder. The case concerns a woman who had rubella in the fifth week of pregnancy, entered the hospital for a therapeutic abortion, and, after a stay of five days, was denied an abortion. Subsequently the child was born with gross abnormalities. This led to a suit against the hospital which was won. If the decision is upheld on constitutional grounds by the Supreme Court, physicians would have to consider the possibility that they might be held liable if they do not perform abortions.

Thus it seems wise, in deciding on tactics, to bear in mind that the objective is not merely to reform the law but to change medical practice. No matter what the law provides, if physicians and hospitals continue to assume that abortions can be done for only a limited number of reasons and, further, that the decision is theirs to make, women will still be forced to turn to the illegal abortionist for this medical procedure, and the movement's victory will be a hollow one. Women living in large metropolitan areas would no doubt find competent medical care but women in small cities and towns (and these are in the majority) might find their situation unchanged.

To be successful, then, the abortion reform movement must not settle for less than the acceptance of abortion as a normal part of medical practice. Anything done to jeopardize that goal is self-defeating.

POSTSCRIPT (OCTOBER, 1970)

As this quick review of what has happened in the past 18 months will show, events are moving very rapidly.

Late in their 1969 legislative sessions, Delaware and Oregon enacted laws based on the ALI Code. Oregon's law, however, goes beyond that model with language taken from the British law, which provides that "In determining whether or not there is substantial risk [to her physical or mental health] account may be taken of the mother's total environment, actual or reasonably foreseeable."

In 1970, the South Carolina and Virginia Legislatures passed, and the governors approved, ALI-type laws. In February 1970, the Hawaii Legislature passed a bill which Governor John A. Burns allowed to become law without his signature. Under this law, any 90-day resident may have an abortion performed by a licensed physician in a licensed hospital if she wants the abortion and a physician agrees to perform the operation. With respect to the residency requirement, the bill states that "The affidavit of such a woman shall be prima facie evidence of compliance with this requirement." Later in 1970, the legislatures of Alaska and New York passed laws similar to the Hawaii law.

In Alaska, Governor Keith Miller vetoed the bill but the legislature overrode his veto. Alaska's new law provides that any 30-day resident can have an abortion (defined as the termination of the "pregnancy of a nonviable fetus") performed by a licensed physician in a hospital or other Health Department-approved facility. New York's law, which was signed by Governor Nelson A. Rockefeller the day after its passage, provides that abortions may be performed by a licensed physician if he believes it is necessary to preserve the patient's life or if the patient is no more than 24 weeks pregnant.

A look at how one of these new laws is working might be useful at this point. As the effective date for New York's law (July 1, 1970) approached, there were the expected predictions of chaos but there was also a good deal of work done by governmental agencies, hospitals, and private groups to prepare to meet the projected demand for this service. Experience in the first two months under the new law indicated that the hard work paid off—the nation's most permissive abortion law was already working reasonably well and the outlook was even better for the future.

New York City's Health Services Administrator, Gordon Chase, reported on September 17, 1970, that between 18,000 and 19,000 abortions had been performed in hospitals. This means that the city's hospitals—municipal, voluntary, and private—were already doing abortions at the rate necessary to meet the estimated demand of some 100,000 a year.

There were four deaths recorded in this early period. One patient died because of adverse reaction to anesthesia; a rheumatic cardiac patient's death was caused by her reaction to the saline solution used in a late abortion; a third patient suffered from sickle-cell anemia; and the fourth died from an infection, possibly caused by an attempted abortion before she entered the hospital.

Converting the city's record of four deaths among 18,000 abortions to the usual health statistic form would give us a figure of 22 deaths per 100,000 abortions. By January 1, 1971, the mortality rate had dropped to eight per 100,000. This compares favorably with England's first year under their new law—21.0 per 100,000—but unfavorably with the countries of Eastern Europe where one to two deaths per 100,000 is the usual rate. Eastern Europe's rate is so low partly because almost no abortions are done after the twelfth week. It is hoped that New York will approach that lower figure by encouraging women to have pregnancy tests early and, if they want abortions, to have them done early.

Since New York's law does not specify where abortions must be done, some (perhaps as many as 5,000) were done, in offices in the early months. However, the New York City Board of Health determined that as of October 19, 1970, abortions would be done only in hospitals, hospital-affiliated clinics, and independent clinics that meet strict specifications as to professional staff, operating-room equipment, blood banks, and laboratory equipment.

While there were those in the abortion reform movement who objected to this as unduly restrictive, others welcomed the move. Since much of the interest in reforming the law has been based specifically on a desire to get the practice of abortion out of offices (and other even less desirable locations) and into hospitals, their approval is not surprising.

While it is much too soon to make a final judgment on how an abortion-on-request law can work in the long run, New York's early experience leads one to be optimistic. Apparently with few exceptions, women—including those without funds—who want abortions can get them in New York City. As more hospital facilities are completed (especially for out-patient abortions) and as more clinics are in operation and as more patients present early in pregnancy, the system should begin to work with what will seem by then to be unremarkable smoothness.

It is encouraging to realize that it need not be all that difficult to make abortion on request work efficiently, since it may well become a national system in the near future. Some state abortion laws have been declared unconstitutional by state and federal district courts and the expectation is that the U.S. Supreme Court will uphold one or more of those decisions when they reach the Court on appeal.

Chapter 3

California's Abortion Law — A Second Look

Edmund W. Overstreet

In 1959 the American Law Institute came forward with a Model Penal Code which recommended the modernization of laws governing abortion. In the same year Packer and Gampell's paper appeared in the May issue of the *Stanford Law Review*, reporting their study of therapeutic abortion *practices* in California, and indicating how greatly these practices had gone beyond the concepts embodied in the California law of that time. Most California physicians were fully aware of these discrepancies, and when the Beilenson bill—which attempted to correct these discrepancies by incorporating the proposals of the American Law Institute—came along, many of us went to work vigorously for its passage. I am sure that all but a very few of us were quite confident that the suggestions of the Model Penal Code, enacted into law, would be almost completely successful in solving the problems we were meeting daily in the practice of therapeutic abortion. Few of us had any notion at that time of the extraordinary and astonishing revolution in attitudes toward abortion which was to take place in the subsequent ten or so years. I must confess that at that time I was an enthusiast for the Model Penal Code as a reasonable solution of our problems, and I can scarcely believe the change in my own thinking that has taken place in the last decade.

Much of that change has come about because of the effects in California of the Therapeutic Abortion Act, which became operative on November 8, 1967. Although it was somewhat emasculated at birth because the provision for fetal indications had been chopped out, it did extend the legal justification for therapeutic abortion to include not only preservation of maternal life, but also when 1) "there is substantial risk that continuance of the pregnancy would gravely impair the physical or mental health of the mother," and when 2) "the pregnancy resulted from rape or incest" (including statutory rape at age 14 or under).

What has happened in California since this law went into effect? First let us simply look at figures. Prior to November, 1967, we have no accurate knowledge of how many therapeutic abortions were being performed in California per year. Various methods of estimation gives us a figure of about 600 per year during the ten years before 1967. This is a rate of 1.8 therapeutic abortions per thousand live births.

Fortunately, we have more dependable knowledge of what is taking place under the Therapeutic Abortion Act, since the State Department of Health is required to query all accredited hospitals in California each year and report the results of the questionnaire to the Legislature. Unfortunately, this procedure has drawbacks in that the reporting by hospitals is voluntary, and the time-lag for individual hospital reports may run to several months. Nevertheless, the available figures present an astounding picture.

During the first calendar year under the new law the number of legal abortions reported from the entire state was 5,030. Only the first six months of 1969 were needed to match this figure, 5,056 being performed. This rapid increase continued unabated so that by the end of 1969 approximately 10,000 more abortions had been performed. While final figures have not yet been published, the California State Department of Health informs me that approximately 24,000 legal abortions were performed during the first six months of 1970. So far, then, the number being performed has doubled every six months. From this trend and other indications, Dr. Edward Jackson of that Department estimates that the figure for the entire year of 1970 will reach 60,000 to 75,000. An increase of 100-fold in only three years under a moderately liberalized law bespeaks the enormous impetus of California women to seek termination of unwanted pregnancies.

Nor has this yet produced its full effect. The State Health Department estimates that at least 40 percent of California women who married under the age of 20 are pregnant at the time, in addition to which there are approximately 40,000 illegitimate births annually. Moreover, it is estimated that of the approximately 354,000 annual births, about one in five are unwanted babies. It has also been fairly reliably estimated that in 1968 approximately 76,000 California women obtained illegal, criminal abortions, in contrast to the 15,000 obtained legally. This sort of information suggests that an estimate of perhaps as many as 150,000 legal abortions in the year 1971 is not an unreasonable one.

As the number of legal abortions increases, the percentage done for reasons of *physical* health continues to decrease—4.9 percent in 1968 and 2.8 percent in 1969. Although this is largely due to the increasing percentage done for *mental* health indications, it also points out the increasingly rare need for abortion as a therapeutic modality when a disease is complicated by pregnancy.

Similarly, the percentage of legal abortions for rape or incest fell from 6.8 percent in 1968 to about 4.5 percent in 1969, but the *actual numbers* remained relatively constant. Under the new law, applications on these grounds must be approved by the county district attorney—an unfortunate delay factor in the committee proceedings. Initially, a small percentage of such applications were turned down by district attorneys, presumably for insufficient prima facie evidence of rape, but after most of these were approved by the subsequent court procedure written into the law, the percentage of district attorney disapproval became very small. In general, district attorneys have taken the attitude that the new law is designed to help victims of rape and incest, not to throw obstacles in their way.

The absence of a fetal indications provision in the new law was, of course, a tragic omission. Opponents of abortion liberalization point to new immunization techniques which may largely remove German measles from the field of indications for therapeutic abortion. But there are several other situations in which delivery of a severely damaged infant may be predicted—notably a series of severely-distorting congenital, hereditary conditions for which no preventive measures are even in prospect. Indeed, a new era in this whole field is just opening up. It is now possible by means of transabdominal puncture and sampling of amniotic fluid before the 16th week of pregnancy to determine the presence of severe *metabolic* disease in the intrauterine infant. This is possible for about ten such diseases at the present time. More and more women are learning about this new possibility and are requesting early diagnosis of such intrauterine fetal disease and therapeutic abortion for it.

This is another example of how a rigid law which incorporates specific indications for therapeutic abortion is in danger of failing to encompass the progress of medical knowledge and public thought.

The fact is that women in general—and certainly California women—are increasingly *unwilling* to accept as offspring the damaged fetuses which a capricious nature occasionally produces. They want to be rid—early in pregnancy—of such mistakes of nature. They are no longer content to produce simply *numbers* of infants; they want to produce the best *quality* of infants of which they are capable. Under the current California law, requests for therapeutic abortion for this reason can only be approved by the subterfuge of threat to the mother's mental health.

The mental health indication now accounts for the great majority of therapeutic abortions being performed—89 percent in 1968 and about 93 percent in 1969. This is the area where we find the greatest furor, the greatest uncertainty among physicians, and great variability in interpretation of the law. The law's actual verbiage is very vague indeed. It speaks of "mental illness to the extent that the woman is dangerous to herself or to the person or property of others or is in need of supervision or restraint." Supervision by whom? A mental hospital? A physician? Friends or family? And how much supervision? Continuous? A daily visit to a psychiatrist? A once a week visit? And when is a woman "dangerous to herself"? Only when she manifests suicidal tendencies? Or is she a danger to herself when she manifests a firm intent to seek *criminal* abortion, with its well-recognized dangers?

Some feel that this vagueness of the law is valuable in that it allows great flexibility of interpretation by individual hospital committees. The trouble is that some hospital committees are very fearful and use this very vagueness to hold down their abortion rates. By contrast, some hospital committees stretch the provisions to encompass what are almost exclusively sociological reasons: unwanted pregnancy; financial stress; marital conflicts; too many children; unmarried pregnancy, etc.

And who is to be the final arbiter in judging whether mental illness is sufficient to justify abortion exists? The California law simply charges the hospital committee with doing so. However, the Joint Commission on Accreditation of Hospitals of the American Medical Association has published guidelines which suggest that when therapeutic abortion is to be carried out "two or more physicians should agree." Traditionally, this has been interpreted as meaning that a patient must have consultation by two psychiatrists. At the present time this type of consultation is usually *in addition to* the adjudication of the case by the hospital committee itself—even though the committee includes psychiatrists among its membership. Obviously a great deal of expense and investment of time—indeed waste of time—is inherent in this procedure. As a result, California psychiatrists are increasingly unhappy with the load of consultations, especially since they concern a matter which many of them find distasteful anyhow. Another difficulty is that some committees avoid the responsibility of making specific judgments about mental illness and simply rubber stamp approval of a patient's application so long as it is accompanied by two affirmative psychiatric consultations. Indeed, committee practices throughout the state vary greatly. Some follow this rubber stamping process; others meet frequently and discuss each case in detail. The latter is an enormous task in view of the mounting number of therapeutic abortions obtained on psychiatric grounds. Nevertheless, there is a trend toward eliminating *any* psychiatric consultant and allowing the patient's physician alone to judge whether "mental illness" exists. This judgment would then be confirmed by the hospital therapeutic abortion committee as required by law.

     As one might expect, the attitudes of hospital committees on what constitutes mental illness vary enormously throughout California. Some hospitals insist that a patient must have shown some evidence of psychiatric illness *before* the start of the current pregnancy in order to be eligible for interruption on psychiatric grounds. This seems utterly illogical to those of us who feel that an inadvertent and unwanted pregnancy—especially in an unstable, unmarried girl—may well be the stress which *first* precipitates significant mental illness. This becomes more likely as the age and marital status pattern of women seeking abortion changes. In California in 1968 only 30 percent of those aborted were married and 53 percent had never been married; by 1969 these figures progressed to 25 percent and 58 percent, respectively. The percentage of those under age 20 climbed from 29 to 32 percent. Clearly, the earlier patterns of *criminal* abortion—over 60 percent for married women with children—do not obtain for *legal* abortion. Indeed, other evidence now suggests that the majority of women who still obtain criminal abortions are also unmarried and in the younger age groups. This has important implications for our concepts about legal "abortion-on-demand"—especially in view of our increasing illegitimacy rates.

Turning now to the racial distribution of abortion patients, we find that ninety percent of therapeutic abortions were performed for white patients and 9 percent for nonwhite patients. This closely corresponds to the racial distribution in California. These figures should help to dispel the notion put forward by racial militants that white physicians are urging and indeed pressuring nonwhite women to have therapeutic abortions and to use contraception in a racially discriminatory fashion—the so-called genocide charge.

Unfortunately, California does not report the religious adherence of abortion patients. However Colorado's experience with its new law reports 17 percent of therapeutic abortion applicants as Catholics as compared to an estimated percentage of Catholics in the state of 22 percent.

How about socioeconomic discrimination? The 40 accredited *county* hospitals in California represent 8.4 percent of the total accredited hospitals and accounted for 9.6 percent of total therapeutic abortions in 1968. But a curious aspect crops up here. Fifty percent of *unmarried* applicants were *disapproved* in county hospitals; less than 7 percent in *private* hospitals. This attitude is not confined to county hospitals. A continuing problem of many hospital committees is the member physician who manifests a punitive attitude toward the results of what he views as illicit sex activity and for this reason he tends to oppose therapeutic abortion for the unmarried teenager more vigorously than for the married mother, even when indications are comparable.

Much of what I have said points to discriminatory aspects of the practice of therapeutic abortion under California's new law. One such aspect seems to be apparent in some of the figures from the first year following its passage; these suggest what might be termed *geographic* discrimination, i.e., marked differences in the geographic distribution of therapeutic abortions being done.

Specifically, there is a major difference in the therapeutic abortion rates of Southern and Northern California. In 1968 the nine San Francisco area counties accounted for 23 percent of California's births; yet 63 percent of California's therapeutic abortions were done there, with a resulting abortion rate of 31 per thousand live births. By contrast, the two counties of the Los Angeles metropolitan area, with 44 percent of the state's births, accounted for only 19 percent of California's therapeutic abortions, with a rate of only 5 per thousand live births. This discrepancy persisted through the first nine months of 1969, but recent establishment of major legal abortion facilities in the Los Angeles area may begin to rectify it. It is difficult to pin down all of the factors which contribute to existing inequities. One of the major ones is the fear on the part of individual hospitals of becoming known as "abortion mills." This is particularly true of smaller rural or suburban hospitals, many of which feel that they do not have the muscle or the prestige to stand up under the possibly critical gaze of the Joint Commission on Accreditation of Hospitals of the American Medical Association. The Joint Commission has specifically disclaimed any intent to regulate abortion rates in such hospitals. For example, in Bulletin #42 (August, 1966) the Commission states that "contrary to occasional rumor, the Joint Commission does not routinely measure the incidence of therapeutic abortion or sterilization procedures carried out in any surveyed hospital against some precise quantitative standard in determining accreditation status." This seemingly straightforward statement would no doubt set hospital fears at rest if the Joint Commission did not go on to contradict itself in the next sentence: "An unusually high proportion of such procedures in the total hospital case load would be given attention." Obviously, the phrase "an unusually high proportion" means that the Joint Commission does think in terms of some incidence limits.

Another factor is the attitudes of patients themselves. Despite the increasing pressure for liberal therapeutic abortion, a degree of social opprobrium still attaches to the woman who has the procedure. This is particularly true for the young unmarried daughter of a "good family" whose pregnancy her family wants to conceal from the local community. These patients tend to apply for therapeutic abortion not at the small, local community hospital but at one of the larger hospitals of a metropolitan area.

Because of these and other factors, the large metropolitan hospitals are being inundated by therapeutic abortion applications. In the ten years before the new law my own hospital averaged ten therapeutic abortions per year—except for a jump in numbers during the rubella epidemic of 1964-65. In 1968 we performed 109 therapeutic abortions for an eleven-fold increase, compared to the state-wide increase of seven-fold. In 1968 our rate was 54 per thousand live births;

at the present time it is approaching 350 per thousand live births. One of the other major San Francisco area hospitals had a rate of approximately 600 abortions per thousand live births during 1969, a rate that rose to about 800 per thousand in 1970.

The failure of the smaller local hospitals to carry their share of the increased load has had an unhappy impact on the functions of the large hospitals, which have had to take up the slack. This is particularly true of the large teaching hospitals, whose training programs and general obstetric-gynecologic services have been materially dislocated by this disproportionately large number of abortion patients. Under the present law this is particularly true of the patients with psychiatric indications because the rigmarole required to adjudicate them is so complex and time-consuming.

The enormously increased patient loads in 1970 have forced resort to a trial of early legal abortion carried out as an outpatient, come-and-go procedure (as is done in the Eastern European countries), even though the state law requires the use of accredited hospital premises. The clamor for having abortions done simply in a medical *office* is mounting, and it will be of great interest to see how this works out in those states whose recently revised laws permit it.

Finally, we come to the question of *economic* discrimination. It has long been said that any woman can obtain an abortion—even a legal one in a hospital—if she can pay for it. This situation is no longer quite as discriminatory as it was before, because under the new law hospitals involved in the care of indigent patients are doing a fair job of carrying their share of the indicated abortions. But economic discrimination does hit the lower middle class American woman who is just above the level of welfare eligibility. Because of the expensive consultation system and the Joint Commission guidelines, the minimal cost to a private patient is about six hundred dollars. And, as always, there are a few physicians who charge whatever the traffic will bear: individual physicians occasionally charge five hundred dollars or more for the procedure to which is added psychiatrists' consultation fees of one hundred dollars or more. It does not speak well of our economic organization of this medical function when one compares these costs with those for equally safe therapeutic abortions in Japan and Eastern Europe. Fortunately, the early experience with outpatient, come-and-go legal abortions suggests that the overall cost can be materially reduced by this approach.

A curious sidelight, which I cannot explain, is seen in the economic attitudes of abortion patients themselves. Even those who are able to afford legal abortion are, in general, rather reluctant to pay the costs of it. Delinquent accounts have been almost the rule. This is so much the case in the San Francisco area that some hospitals now insist on an admission deposit of about four hundred dollars for abortion patients, and some physicians will not even accomplish initial office examination of such patients without a preliminary deposit of about two hundred dollars, returnable if the hospital committee disapproves the procedure. One might wonder whether this psychological quirk of patients is related to the emphasis on therapeutic abortion as primarily a *legal* matter which principally concerns the state rather than as an integral part of medical care. Perhaps this attitude is further reflected in the growing public expression (by women's liberation groups, for example) that legal abortion-on-demand ought to be available to *all* women *without cost.*

At the time that California's half-hearted liberalization of the law was fought through the legislature there were a few who supported it on the grounds that it would contribute significantly to the solution of the problem of criminal abortion. Most of us felt that this was a false emphasis and that the new law would have very little impact upon this problem. Subsequent events have shown both groups to be partly right. Obviously, the 5,030 legal abortions in 1968 scarcely made a dent in the estimated yearly 75,000 to 100,000 criminal abortions. But sixty thousand or so legal abortions in 1970 would undoubtedly materially reduce their number. That this is already happening is strongly suggested by a recent (unpublished) study of abortion patients at the San Francisco General Hospital (1). Since advent of the new law the incidence of septic abortion patients (presumably criminally induced) has steadily and rapidly decreased. The same decrease is being seen in abortion-related maternal deaths, formerly the greatest single cause of maternal death in California. And for the first time in the history of that hospital there were *no* deaths from that cause in 1969!

It is in this area—that of criminal abortion—that we deal almost entirely with the problem of pregnancies which are simply desperately *unwanted* for purely socioeconomic reasons. Unfortunately, the restrictions of the new law are not well understood by California women. Physicians are seeing more and more patients who demand interruption of pregnancy not on legal grounds but simply because they want to be rid of an inadvertent, unexpected, unplanned-for, totally unwanted pregnancy.

They come also for this motive after the failure of contraception. They argue quite reasonably: "You were perfectly willing to give me medical care to help me prevent any further pregnancies; why won't you give me an abortion now that your own medical prescription has failed?" Indeed, this reveals a surprisingly widespread inadequacy in the actual prescription of contraceptive methods to California women. Many of these failures of birth control are the result of poor understanding of the method employed due to inadequate instruction by the prescribing physician.

If the estimate of 150,000 legal abortions in California in 1971 is even approached, it seems clear that criminal abortion will become relatively rare. In addition, the figure will include many pregnancies resulting from failed contraception, as well as an increasing number which are unwanted for socioeconomic reasons.

At the present time the entire problem of unwanted pregnancy is undergoing thorough medical review. Psychiatrists are increasingly of the opinion that forcing a woman to bear an *unwanted* child almost inevitably results in harm to her mental health and to that of her child. Recent studies from Sweden(2) suggest this very strongly and careful investigation of this proposition is under way in the United States. If confirmed, it would have obvious implications for the current California law because approval of therapeutic abortion would then depend only upon a judgment as to whether a pregnancy is truly *unwanted*. Indeed, one suspects that this type of interpretation is implicit in the skyrocketing abortion rate; many of the abortions now being done are simply for unwanted pregnancy.

Meanwhile the pressure for repeal of all abortion statutes is growing with astonishing speed. What is important is that women in general are making their views more vigorously heard as the important principals in this issue. Increasingly they claim the decision of the U.S. Supreme Court in *Griswold v. Connecticut*(3) as a manifesto which gives to the individual woman the right to avoid childbearing, even though abortion be involved. The example of Great Britain, which has a provision for socioeconomic and environmental indications in its new law, is no doubt a factor in the reform movement. As a result, the numbers of therapeutic abortions in Great Britain are increasing by leaps and bounds. Recently the chief of the University of Cambridge,

England, maternity hospital informed me that their rate is running at approximately 200 abortions per 1,000 live births and that they have established a separate 12-bed unit in the hospital expressly for these patients. He noted the existence of charter plan flights from the continent of Europe to England for the purpose of bringing women who want to be rid of unwanted pregnancies. Clearly, this world-wide trend for what Professor Garrett Hardin calls "the abolition of compulsory pregnancy" is gaining extraordinary force.

In my opinion there is no doubt whatever that the *legal* restrictions which stand in the way of abortion-on-request will soon be removed. A major impetus for this is inherent in the population explosion. All of us increasingly feel its dire impact in our daily lives, and we are slowly beginnning to recognize the desperate necessity for the reduction of birth rates. We in California feel it perhaps more strongly, with the state's population increasing by about 10,000 *per week*. Even now population limitation is still regarded as a matter for individual, voluntary, family planning. However, as Professor Kingsley Davis points out, the likelihood that voluntary birth control alone can accomplish actual population control is almost nil. For those concerned with this problem, I think his paper in the 10 November, 1967, issue of *Science* should be rewarding reading. Davis reminds us that family planning programs have so far failed to demonstrate any ability to lower birth rates significantly, whereas elective, induced abortion "is one of the surest means of controlling reproduction, and one that has been *proved* capable of reducing birth rates rapidly." He goes on to emphasize the irony of the situation when those most ardently advocating family planning and population control deny the central tenet of their own movement by decrying legalization of elective abortion. But a few more years of watching the quality of our human living steadily downgraded by the population explosion will, I think, convince us that elective abortion must become an accepted practice in the United States, as it is in other parts of the world.

REFERENCES

1. Stewart, G. and Goldstein, P. Therapeutic abortion in California: Effects on septic abortion and maternal mortality. (To be published in *Obstetrics and Gynecology*)
2. Forssman, H. and Thuwe, T. One hundred and twenty children born after application for therapeutic abortion refused. *Acta Psychiat. Scand. 42:*71, 1966. See Appendix A.
3. Griswold v. Connecticut, 381 U.S. 479, 481 (1965).

Chapter **4**

Grounds
for
Legal Challenge

Norma G. Zarky

NOTE: This chapter has been adapted from a paper delivered to The California Committee on Therapeutic Abortion Conference in May, 1969. At that time, not even the landmark case of *People v. Belous*, 71 Cal. 2d 954, 458 P. 2d 194, 80 Cal. Rptr. 354 (1969), cert. denied, 397 U.S. 915 (1970) (holding unconstitutional the California law in existence prior to 1967) had been decided. In the intervening period, the grounds for legal challenge itemized and discussed in this chapter have been utilized in cases far too numerous to mention. No attempt is made here to discuss the results of any single case, or to comment on existing decisions. The law with respect to the validity of various forms of anti-abortion statutes has moved so quickly and will probably have developed so much during the period of publication of this book that any review of the status of cases would be more appropriate in a periodical publication. The major cases decided prior to October, 1970, are listed in Chapter 5 by Ruth Roemer, at page 39 of this text.

Although the abortion laws had their genesis around the middle of the 1800's, and have long been described as "antiquated," their validity has only recently been challenged in the courts. Up until the fall of 1968, no cases involving full-scale attack upon a state abortion law had been brought in the United States. Perhaps this has not been due to the fact that the primary constitutional issues which are raised by the abortion law challenges are expressed in "antiquated" constitutional principles, but because they have only recently received recognition and emphasis. However, the development of our current concepts of woman's individual rights and the right of privacy under constitutional law, has been accompanied by the development of the view that a challenge of the abortion laws through the courts is possible and inevitable. This is truly an issue whose time has come.

An accepted principle of our constitutional law is that constitutional concepts are not static and must be examined in the light of current knowledge(1). Time and time again, our concepts of a

27

constitutional right have changed; in our generation, perhaps the most significant example of this was the overturning of the separate but equal doctrine in the area of education and elsewhere.

BASES FOR CHALLENGE TO RESTRICTIVE STATE ABORTION LAWS

The Statutes Violate a Fundamental Right of Women

The fault of the state abortion statutes lies in their refusal to recognize the right of a woman to determine the number of offspring she will bear, or, as others phrase it, the right of a woman to control her reproductive function. This is the essential underlying constitutional theory upon which all state action restricting abortions (except such minimal action as may be required by the state's proper control of the practice of medicine) must be challenged. Other constitutional attacks discussed in this chapter—those arising from the form of statutory language or the unequal bearing of the statute on various classes of women—can, if successful, result in revised, more carefully framed abortion statutes which would give due regard to equality in application, but which would still restrict the woman's individual freedom. The real thrust of a constitutional challenge, if it is to result in effective restraint upon anti-abortion laws, must lie in the concept of woman's fundamental rights as delineated above. That concept has not yet received explicit recognition in the United States Supreme Court(2). However, recognition of a woman's right to control her own body has been foreshadowed by a long line of cases going back to the last century, in which numerous related personal rights, such as a "right to raise a family," a "right to marry," a "right to have offspring," and the "right of parents to direct the upbringing of their children" have been treated as having constitutionally protected status. Certainly, each of the personal rights so recognized and protected would seem to be of less essential importance to those concepts of human dignity and equality which should govern the constitutional protection of individual freedoms than woman's basic right which is invaded by our state abortion statutes.

Support for this argument may be found in the United States Supreme Court's relatively recent recognition in *Griswold v. Connecticut*(3) of a constitutional "right to privacy" which the Court described as being "older than the Bill of Rights." This was primarily the basis on which the Court held the anti-contraceptive statute of Connecticut to be unconstitutional. The right to privacy is not specifically enumerated in the Bill of Rights. However, it is one that has been added by the Supreme Court to the list of those specifically enumerated in the Constitution and which demand the same degree of protection against state interference as those included in the Bill of Rights.

Important to the challenge based upon unwarranted invasion of a woman's fundamental personal right is a documentation of the extent to which the vaunted personal freedom is recognized by the community. Representatives of virtually every important segment of society have indicated their recognition and acceptance of a personal right to make decisions regarding the bearing of children. Among them are the American Public Health Association, medical organizations, the Citizens Advisory Council on the Status of Women, the Section of Family Law of the American Bar Association, the President's Task Force on the Administration of Justice and, with the exception of the Catholic Church, the major religious groups in the United States.

Some analysts urge the position that there are two separate constitutional rights involved: 1. the right of a woman to determine the size of her family; and 2. the right of privacy. This may not be a meaningful distinction, since the legal arguments are based upon virtually the same cases as precedents. There are also those who think that there may be a distinct right of "marital privacy" based on certain language in the *Griswold* case. However, in whatever direction one shapes the argument or describes the nature of the invaded right, the most important challenge to a restrictive abortion law would be based upon the invasion of woman's personal freedom.

The Statutes Violate a Fundamental Right of Physicians

The invasion of the right of physicians to give medical advice and treatment in accordance with their professional knowledge is also a ground for challenge of the laws which permit punishment of all, including physicians, who perform abortions. In every action in which a doctor is prosecuted for performing or aiding in an abortion, the constitutionality of the statute which he is alleged to have violated can be challenged. The same issues may be raised by actions that are brought by physicians, either personally or on behalf of all physicians who practice in the field of obstetrics and gynecology, to have state abortion laws declared invalid. Any law which, in effect, restricts a physician from performing abortions where indicated, inhibits and curtails the proper practice of medicine. The physician's interest in his own freedom to advise his patients, in the light of his best professional knowledge, as to their medical needs for treatment, has already been clearly recognized in the Connecticut contraceptive cases and in certain prior federal cases.

Because constitutional challenges can be based either on the invasion of woman's fundamental right or the restriction of the physician's right just described, it is relevant to mention the procedural relationship between these two rights in actions involving an attack on the abortion laws.

A physician can obviously raise the issue of the violation of his own constitutional rights in every case in which he is involved. However, it is significant for planning the strategy of constitutional challenges that a physician also has the right, under a doctrine well-established, to assert the constitutional rights of other persons affected. Thus, the basic constitutional question of woman's rights can be raised and discussed in cases involving only physicians as plaintiffs or defendants. This useful legal principle permits physicians of standing and prominence to bring actions, not only on behalf of other doctors similarly situated, but to use their attack to assert the rights of the woman.*

The Ancillary Argument — There is No Sufficient State Interest Requiring Restriction of the Fundamental Rights of Women and/ or of Physicians

Recognition and establishment of the fundamental rights of women or of physicians which we have outlined do not, in themselves, resolve the constitutional issue. If there is a sufficient state interest, a constitutional right may be invaded and statutes that restrict the exercise of that right are valid, despite the invasion. Therefore, the

*In numerous cases brought since this paper was presented, the technique mentioned has been utilized. Other actions have been brought solely on behalf of women plaintiffs, as a class or as individuals. This may present timing difficulties if the woman plaintiff is already pregnant and is asking immediate relief.

asserted interest must be examined and its importance compared with the fundamental nature of the right one seeks to protect.

Accordingly, in each instance in which an anti-abortion law is challenged, it becomes necessary to show that there is no interest which justifies the challenged invasion. This should involve a specific negation of each possible ground, and a factual demonstration that the interest either does not exist, or that it is not of sufficient strength to justify the invasion of the constitutionally protected right.

One other legal principle that should be mentioned is, in a way, related to the issue of sufficient state interest. This principle, frequently described as the "overbreadth" doctrine, requires that an invasion of personal constitutional rights, even if supported by a state interest, must be restricted as narrowly as possible in the light of the evils which it is designed to prevent.

The alleged health interest.   A state may claim that the protection of woman's health requires the kind of restrictions on abortion that are embodied in the typical abortion law. While this may have been true at the time most of these laws were passed, the advances in antisepsis and surgical procedures have been so great that the reverse can now be demonstrated. Statistics reveal that the possibility of death from childbirth now exceeds the possibility of death from an abortion performed by a licensed physician in an antiseptic setting. Moreover, the unavailability of legal, safe abortions has created a major public health problem. The great number of abortions performed in inappropriate, unclean surroundings and by untrained persons has led to wide incidence of severe infection and permanent physical damage. The so-called "health argument" on behalf of the state can be made to backfire by showing to the courts the urgent health problems which the unrealistic state laws have brought about.

The sexual promiscuity argument.   Proponents of strict abortion laws often argue that the control of sexual promiscuity and immoral acts requires state interference with the availability of abortion. This argument is not often or strongly made in formal statements of the state's position, however, possibly because of its patent invalidity. There is no evidence that varying degrees of sexual freedom are in any way related to the availability of abortions; rather, they relate to changing social mores. Indeed, it should be emphasized that it is the married woman, equally or more often than the college girl or unmarried career woman, who seeks an illegal abortion, or a legal one where this is available, thus indicating that the problem is not at all one of sexual promiscuity.

In fact, even if it were (in whole or in part) the evil which the abortion laws were designed to meet, the statutes would still be subject to the claim of overbreadth and the prohibitions of these laws should be tailored so as to deal only with that evil. For example, in a statue narrowly addressed to the "promiscuity" evil, prohibitions should not apply to married women, women who have a one-person relationship, or women in any similar classes.

The state's need for population expansion. This is another argument which history has rendered totally impotent. In the face of the present population explosion, no persuasive argument can be made on the part of the State that restrictive abortion laws are required in order to ensure adequate population.

The alleged "Rights of the Fetus." The state interest most frequently advanced in support of present anti-abortion laws is the theoretical right of the state to protect an embryonic spark of life from destruction. This argument is most noticeably urged by members of religious groups which presently take the position that life begins at conception. It is rebutted by the lack of historical evidence to indicate that the legislatures had such protection in mind when they passed the 19th century anti-abortion statutes. Indeed, as has been noted earlier, the available evidence indicates that the state interest at that time was in protecting women from the health dangers inherent in pre-antiseptic surgery.

Advocates of the "right to life" concept support it by citing cases in which certain rights of the unborn have been recognized in the areas of property laws and tort laws. Those cases are distinguishable, for in nearly every instance, the protection was granted to a viable fetus or one which was subsequently born alive, or it was a right of the parents rather than the fetus. Regardless of such technical points, cases decided in an area in which the mother's and fetus' needs and desires are identical, offer no guide and no precedent for a holding that the state can properly give precedence to a piece of protoplasm over a full-grown living human being. For those to whom a piece of protoplasm and a full-grown person are of equal value, no abortion is required, but their religious and philosophical views cannot confer validity on statutes that require those who feel otherwise to bear and rear a child.

Most of the State Statutes are Vague and Indefinite and,
Therefore, Invalid

The vast majority of jurisdictions in the United States permit abortions only when "necessary for the preservation of the mother's life." Also, one of our accepted constitutional principles (applied with particular care to criminal statutes) is that a statute must give warnings of what acts to do so it is unconstitutionally vague. Within this "void for vagueness" doctrine, many state anti-abortion statutes are almost certainly invalid. For example does the statutory language mean life only in the sense of not being dead, or in the sense of the quality of life as that term is used by doctors and sociologists today? Does it mean that the chances of a pregnant woman's dying must be 100 percent, 80 percent, or only just over 50 percent? The extent (as shown by social studies) to which hospital authorities and doctors vary in their application of the doctrine of "void for vagueness" confirms the uncertainty of the statutory language.

When states have attempted to interpret this language in particular cases, the decisions have also been so confusing that they have not provided the doctor with any real line of demarcation between facts which would surely satisfy the statutory standard and facts which would fall outside its ambit. Thus the doctor, who is criminally liable for any mistakes in judgment, if left with no choice but to engage in the kind of guesswork which, in most cases, will lead him to decide against an abortion. The vagueness of the statute results in an impingement on woman's fundamental rights in addition to presenting an unfair choice to physicians.

The challenge based on the particular language of the statutes may be adopted by the courts more readily than the arguments set forth as to woman's and the physician's rights for the very reason that it does not require the court to confront the more fundamental constitutional issue. However, as mentioned earlier, a decision voiding a statute on the grounds of vague statutory language will permit a state legislature to attempt to structure a statute with more appropriate and clearly defined terms and will result in a postponement of a definitive constitutional decision. From the point of view of those challenging the statutes, a decision on the "void for vagueness" ground would be a tactical but not a strategic victory.

Unequal Application of the Laws

Restrictive abortion laws may be challenged on the grounds that they are discriminatory, both on their face and in their application. Again, the constitutional principle is clear—a state statute which, without rational basis, invidiously discriminates among classes of persons violates the fourteenth amendment to the United States Constitution. On the face of it, the typical "preservation of life" statute discriminates against the following classes of women:

    a.   Women who are healthy;

    b.   Women who are not healthy, but whose health problems are not of such seriousness as to require a medical finding that an abortion is necessary to preserve her life;

    c.   Women whose contraceptive methods failed;

    d.   Women who are raped;

    e.   Women who, (because of their exposure to rubella or drugs, or for such other reasons as hereditary factors), are faced with the probability of bearing a defective child.

Such patent discrimination can only be upheld if there is clear justification for it. That there is no such justification is shown by our foregoing examination of the alleged grounds of state interest.

A more difficult challenge to support is that based upon the application, in practice, of the presently existing anti-abortion laws to different classes of women. An attack based upon this challenge requires detailed factual documentation. We tend to accept as a fact that the laws are discriminatory in their application, that they favor one class of women over another, i.e., the rich or moderately well-to-do, sophisticated, white woman over the disadvantaged minority-group woman. Whether courts will take judicial notice of that social situation, without further evidence, is highly debatable. Fortunately, studies carried out by sociologists and other researchers have resulted in the compilation of data that demonstrates the existence of the general discrimination described above:

    a.   A greater proportion of abortions are performed in private than in public hospitals; thus the woman who has access to a private hospital is favored.

b.   Non-white women receive fewer abortions, proportionately, than white women.

c.   The incidence of severe infection and death (associated with abortion) among poor women or women of minority ethnic groups is very much higher than that of middle-class white women.

Many of these studies are, naturally, a few years old and were limited in geographical areas covered. In a particular state, results of the studies may be only of indirect use because they deal with practices in another jurisdiction. Therefore, a well-prepared argument on this issue would be most useful if it included the most recent statistical material available from the particular jurisdiction. Those preparing legal challenges may, therefore, in some instances be well advised to support the funding and carrying out of local studies that cover time periods as close to the time of filing the case as possible. Sometimes the state health statistics will be of assistance in this area. It must be reemphasized that a challenge based on the ground of unequal application of the law is most likely—perhaps only likely—to be successful when it is based on detail, rather than on generalizations which many who are concerned with the abortion problem believe to be true, but which have not always been documented.

The Establishment of Religion Argument

It has been suggested that an additional ground for challenge of the anti-abortion statutes in that they violate the First Amendment provision which prohibits laws respecting an establishment of religion or the free exercise thereof (generally referred to as the doctrine of separation of church and state). Of course, the First Amendment is, on its face, a restriction only upon the activities of Congress. However, by virtue of a series of cases, most of the principles of the Bill of Rights, including the prohibition against establishment of religion, have been applied to state as well as federal action.

Thus, whenever the purpose or primary effect of a legislative enactment is the advancement or inhibition of a religious dogma, that enactment is unconstitutional. It may be possible, in a particular factual situation, to demonstrate that the activities of a particular religious group have affected the course of legislative enactment to the end that the anti-abortion laws of a state are maintained solely for the reason that they do not contravene the tenets of that group. In my opinion, it is not enough to show that the philosophy of a restrictive abortion law corresponds with the dogma of a particular group, but it must also be shown that the purpose or primary effect of the statute is the maintenance of the dogma. An example of the kind of case in which the Supreme Court will find such primary purpose or effect is the decision that struck down the Tennessee statute which embodied the fundamentalist theory of evolution and prohibited the teaching of the Darwinian theory. If a sufficient showing can be made that a particular state statute restricting abortion laws was either (1) initially passed or (2) retained against attack, primarily to effectuate a religious dogma, it may be possible to challenge the law on this additional ground.

CONCLUSION

Growing concern over restrictive abortion laws has generated nationwide interest in legal challenges to such laws. Regardless of the outcome of any particular challenge to any particular state law, one or more of those briefly outlined here should have sufficient thrust to bring about the invalidation of a substantial number of existing state laws.

Of course, a clear ruling by the United States Supreme Court, holding an abortion law unconstitutional on broad constitutional grounds (that is, invasion of the physician's and/or woman's right) would, for all practical purposes, settle the issue for all the states. The Supreme Court can avoid such a ruling by its power to restrict those cases on which it rules, or by choosing a limited ground on which to base a ruling. The latter course would be in the tradition of the judicial self-restraint which leads a court to decide a case involving constitutional law on the narrowest, rather than the broadest, possible grounds. Were such a decision to be made, the result would probably be a diversity of state rulings that would exist for years.

REFERENCES

1. Harper v. Virginia State Board of Elections, 383 U.S. 663, 86 S.Ct. 1079 (1966), at 383 U.S. 669.
2. At the time of publication of this book, although not at the time of

the giving of this paper, the Supreme Court of California had, in the *Belous* case, distinctly recognized such a right in the woman, and this aspect of the *Belous* opinion had been followed by many courts. See Appendix B.

3. Griswold v. Connecticut, 381 U.S. 479, 85 S.Ct. 1678 (1965).

Chapter 5

Abortion Law Reform and Repeal: Legislative and Judicial Developments

Ruth Roemer

In the three years from 1967 to 1970, a revolution has occurred in the abortion laws and practices in the United States. That revolution is still in process. Our once highly restrictive anti-abortion laws have been reformed in 13 states and virtually repealed in four states. No other country has a statute which explicitly makes abortion a matter for decision by the woman and her physician. Although other countries permit abortion on request of the woman under certain circumstances, the four American states have pioneered in treating abortion, as a matter of law, like any other medical procedure.

As a result of recent developments, the United States has become a laboratory in which three different types of legal regulation of abortion can be compared and evaluated.* We can also profit from the longer experience of other countries with abortion statutes of varying liberality, although account must be taken of differing family planning programs and systems of delivering health services.

Presented to Panel on Abortion, Section on Maternal and Child Health, American Public Health Association Convention, Houston, Texas, October 29, 1970.

*Acknowledgments: For helpful information on recent legal cases, grateful acknowledgment is made to four authorities on abortion law: Roy Lucas, Norma Zarky, Alan Charles, and Zad Leavy. Any errors are, of course, the responsibility of the author.

LEGISLATIVE DEVELOPMENTS IN THE UNITED STATES

Three kinds of modernized abortion laws have been enacted in the United States since 1967: 1. Twelve states have enacted all or part of the Model Penal Code first proposed in 1957 by the American Law Institute (ALI), under which abortion is not a crime when performed by a licensed physician because of substantial risk that continuance of the pregnancy would gravely impair the physical or mental health of the woman or that the child would be born with grave physical or mental defect, or in cases of pregnancy resulting from rape or incest(1). 2. One state, Oregon, has expanded the American Law Institute grounds to include a sociomedical ground proposed originally by the American College of Obstetricians and Gynecologists(2) and patterned after a provision of the British Abortion Act of 1967(3), i.e., that in determining whether or not there is substantial risk to the woman's physical or mental health, account may be taken of her total environment, actual or reasonably foreseeable(4). 3. Four states— Alaska(5), Hawaii(6), New York(7), and the State of Washington (by referendum in November 1970)—have repealed all criminal penalties for abortion provided only that the abortion is done early in pregnancy and by a licensed physician (Alaska, Hawaii, and Washington also stipulate that the operation must take place in a licensed hospital or other approved facility). Thirty-three states, however, still have laws making abortion a crime except when performed to save the life (or, in a few instances, the health) of the woman. None of these states even requires that the abortion be performed by a licensed physician.

The details of the new laws and their varying provisions are summarized in Table 1. The key developments relate to six general aspects:

1. All 17 states require that the abortion be performed by a licensed physician.

2. All the states with new laws, except Mississippi and New York,* require that the abortion be performed in hospitals, with Kansas also permitting another place designated by law(8).

*New York City has recently added the requirement that abortions be performed in hospitals or clinics, and not in doctors' offices. The State of Washington requires that abortions be performed in accredited hospitals or approved medical facilities.

3.   All 17 states allow abortion to save the life of the woman, and also in pregnancies resulting from sex crimes.

All these 17 states (except Mississippi, which authorizes abortion only for rape or to save life) allow abortion to preserve the health or the physical or mental health of the woman. The sociomedical standard of the Oregon law mentioned above is a broader standard than the medical standard of the ALI-style laws.

Seven states set age limits on abortions for statutory rape. These limits may be lower than the age of consent. Thus, in California sexual intercourse with an unmarried girl below the age of 18 constitutes statutory rape; but if pregnancy results, it can be terminated only if the girl is below the age of 15.

All 17 states, except California and Mississippi, allow abortion for fetal abnormality.

4.   The maximum time limits within which abortions may be performed vary from 16 weeks in Colorado, New Mexico, and Washington to 26 weeks in Maryland. In Oregon the time limit is 150 days. In Alaska and Hawaii, the fetus must be nonviable. In New York the time limit is 24 weeks.

5.   Medical approval by consultants, boards, or hospital therapeutic abortion committees is required in all states (except Mississippi) with ALI-style laws, although the Model Penal Code did not propose such procedures. In Oregon, two physicians must certify the circumstances justifying an abortion. In Alaska, Hawaii, and New York, only one physician is required.

6.   New York and the following ALI-style states have no residency requirement: California, Colorado, Kansas, Maryland, Mississippi, and New Mexico. South Carolina, Hawaii, and the State of Washington have a 90-day residency requirement, and Arkansas, Delaware, North Carolina, and Virginia require four months' residency. Oregon requires that the patient be a resident. Alaska requires a 30 days' residency.

Actual practice, of course, may differ from the provisions of the statutes. In some places, doctors will not perform abortions as late as the statute allows. Nonresidents may not be welcomed even though the state has no residency requirement. Consents, consultations, and committee approvals may be required that are not specified in the statutes. It is also possible that residency requirements may not be strictly enforced and procedures may be more simple than those provided in the statute.

On the federal level, a bill introduced in Congress by Senator Packwood to legalize abortion throughout the nation made no progress. A recent policy enunciated for U.S. military hospitals, however, permits abortions and sterilizations for military personnel, active or retired, and their families, regardless of state or local laws(9). In October, 1970, a White House task force on the mentally handicapped recommended that, in the interest of both maternal and child mental health, no woman should be forced to bear an unwanted child.

JUDICIAL DEVELOPMENTS IN THE UNITED STATES

Legislative developments have been accompanied by an emerging body of court decisions on the constitutionality of anti-abortion laws. The picture changes almost from day to day. As of autumn 1970, five cases were on the U.S. Supreme Court docket, more than 20 cases were before three-judge federal courts; and, excluding the 20 states with federal cases, many of which also had state cases, another 11 states had cases pending in local courts(10). The following important cases may be noted.

1. In September, 1969, the Supreme Court of California, in the first decision on the constitutionality of any anti-abortion statute, invalidated the pre-1967 anti-abortion law of California. In a four to three decision in *People v. Belous*(11), the court held the statute unconstitutional on two principal grounds: 1. that the phrase, "necessary to preserve life," was so vague as to be violative of the due process requirements for a criminal law, and 2. that the law was in violation of a woman's fundamental rights to life and to choose whether to bear children. The latter follows from the U.S. Supreme Court's acknowledgment of a right of privacy or liberty in matters related to marriage, family, and sex(12).

The critical issue defined by the California Supreme Court was whether the state had any legitimate interest in the regulation of abortion which would justify so deep an infringement of the fundamental rights of women. The court held that the state had no such compelling interest. The court said that it would not speak to the constitutionality of the current California Therapeutic Abortion Act, since Dr. Belous was charged under the old law. But one might well infer from the decision that the current law may be declared unconstitutional on similar grounds. The court did express the view, however, that the decision to terminate pregnancy under the 1967 Therapeutic Abortion Act was solely a medical one, and so long as the physician follows the procedural requirements of the Act his judgment may not later be challenged by a jury or prosecutor in a criminal case.

2.   Following the landmark decision of the California Supreme Court, the first decision of a federal court invalidating an anti-abortion statute was handed down. In *U.S. v. Vuitch*(13), the U.S. District Court for the District of Columbia held unconstitutional the District of Columbia statute which made abortion a felony unless performed by a licensed physician for the preservation of the mother's life or health. The court held this phrase so uncertain and ambiguous as to invalidate the statute for want of due process, and it recommended appeal to the U.S. Supreme Court. The opinion of Judge Gerhard A. Gesell in *Vuitch* emphasized, as the *Belous* decision had done, the woman's liberty and right of privacy in matters related to family, marriage, and sex and the necessity for demonstrating affirmatively the interest of the state in infringing on such rights. The opinion pointed out the discriminatory application of the statute with respect to women who are poor. This case is now on appeal to the U. S. Supreme Court, which has raised certain jurisdictional questions concerning the propriety of direct appeal to the Supreme Court without first proceeding to the U. S. Court of Appeals for the District of Columbia.

3.   In addition to these two decisions which broke new legal ground, a number of other courts have invalidated pre-ALI-style anti-abortion laws. These cases have arisen in both federal and state courts.

Three-judge panels of federal district courts have held the pre-ALI-style laws of Texas(14) and Wisconsin(15) unconstitutional because of overbreadth. One court also held the statute void for vagueness, and both courts found the statutes an unconstitutional invasion of private rights and not justified by a compelling interest of the state. Contrary is one federal court which, in a two to one decision, upheld the anti-abortion statute of Louisiana(16).

Similar suits have been brought in federal courts involving the Arizona(17), Illinois(18), and New Jersey laws(19). Suits challenging the Kentucky(20) and Minnesota(21) laws were dismissed on jurisdictional grounds, and the New York case was dismissed as moot on repeal of New York's anti-abortion statute(22).

State courts have also struck down pre-ALI-style laws. In Illinois, a judge of the criminal court held the abortion statute unconstitutional on grounds of vagueness and infringement on the woman's right to control her body(23). In Pennsylvania, a county court judge found that the state's statute impinges on constitutionally protected areas and is so broad, unlimited, and indiscriminate that it fails to meet present-day tests for constitutionality(24). In South Dakota, a circuit court condemned the statute because it interferes with private conduct without serving any vital interest of society(25). In Michigan, the statute was found defective as infringing on the right of privacy in the physician-patient relationship and as possibly violative of the patient's right to safe and adequate medical treatment(26). Contra, however, is the Massachusetts Supreme Judicial Court, which upheld the constitutionality of the state's statute prohibiting "unlawful" abortion against a charge of vagueness in a case sustaining revocation of a medical license(27). Suits challenging other pre-ALI-style laws are still pending elsewhere(28).

4. Attempts are currently being made to obtain an adjudication of the constitutionality of reformed ALI-style laws(29). Thus far, only one reformed ALI-style law has been invalidated by a federal court— Georgia's 1968 abortion law. The U.S. District Court in Atlanta held unconstitutional those parts of the 1968 Georgia law that limited the woman's right to abortion to the three ALI grounds(30). The basis of the court's decision was violation of the woman's right of privacy. Retained as a proper exercise of state power, however, were the requirements for medical consultation, hospital committee approval, hospital accreditation and exemption provisions, and the residency requirement.

On the state level, the California Therapeutic Abortion Act has been challenged in three cases. Two cases involving Doctors Robb and Gwynne are still pending, but preliminary decisions involving these doctors have held the California statute unconstitutional(31). In *People v. Barksdale*, a municipal court in Alameda County held the current California law unconstitutional as violative of the equal protection clause of the 14th Amendment, as a vague and improper delegation of legislative authority to the Joint Commission on Accreditation of Hospitals, as discriminatory between the rich and the poor, as lacking the certainty required for a criminal statute with respect to the definition of mental illness, and as violative of the fundamental right of the woman to make a free choice whether or not to bear children(32). In rejecting the argument that the state has a compelling interest in protecting the embryo, Judge T. L. Foley added the following poignant words:

> I might say that I belong to the religion that was just referred to, and I dislike to render this opinion. I must follow the law under my oath as a Judge. I am a Catholic which makes it very, very difficult—but my oath of office calls for me to follow the law as stated and set out by the Appellate Courts of this State(33).

The judicial picture is in constant flux as new cases are filed in federal and state courts; as the defense of unconstitutionality is raised in criminal prosecutions of doctors; as issues are raised concerning jurisdiction of courts and standing of plaintiffs to sue; and as decisions come down and appeals are taken.

On at least eight occasions, the United States Supreme Court has declined to review state court decisions that involved restrictive anti-abortion laws(34). One of these cases was the landmark decision of the California Supreme Court in *Belous*. On October 13, 1970, the Court dismissed an appeal from the decision of a three-judge federal court holding the Wisconsin anti-abortion statute unconstitutional(35). Action by the Court on the merits of abortion cases will be decisive, but it is possible that some of the cases will go off on questions of jurisdiction or on grounds other than the basic constitutional issues.

Although the final outcome cannot be predicted, three eventualities seem fairly certain. First, more and more states will change their laws in accordance with one or another of the three patterns now prevailing in the United States. Second, as in other nations of the world, moderately reformed laws will be amended to expand the grounds and to simplify the procedures; alternatively, anti-abortion laws will be repealed. Third, in every state pressure will mount for making abortion available *de facto* as well as *de jure* to women, rich and poor, faced with the despair and desperation occasioned by unwanted pregnancy.

RECENT DEVELOPMENTS IN OTHER COUNTRIES

The abortion laws of the world have been described on a five-stage continuum, ranging from the most permissive to the most restrictive(36). Recent legislative changes show that more and more countries are liberalizing their laws or the interpretation of their laws all along this continuum.

Abortion on the Insistence of the Woman

No new jurisdictions have joined this category, except the four states in the United States discussed above. The tightening of the Bulgarian law in 1968(37) in order to encourage population growth has been eased by a 1970 interpretation that allows abortion virtually on request for unmarried women and women having at least one child(38). The hope is that this interpretation will reduce the number of illegal abortions. In these cases, the Bulgarian law resembles once again the most liberal laws of the USSR and Hungary. Now that the German Democratic Republic has liberalized its policy on abortion, as mentioned below, the only restrictive abortion statutes remaining in eastern Europe are those of Romania and Albania.

Abortion on Social Grounds

Two Scandinavian countries, Finland and Denmark, have liberalized their statutes further to include social grounds. The 1970 law in Finland specifies, in addition to medical and humanitarian reasons and the age of the mother (under 17 or over 40 or already the mother of four children), the following social ground:

> when the delivery and care of the child would constitute, by reason of the conditions of existence of the woman and her family, as well as other circumstances, a change for her(39).

A unique provision, relevant for all countries faced with expanding demand for abortions, requires the Finnish Department of Health to assure a sufficient number of qualified physicians and abortion hospitals and also impartial and uniform conduct from physicians.

The Danish law of 1970 permits abortion without authorization of a committee for reasons of life or health or in cases where the woman is over 38 or has four children under age 18 who reside with her(40). Authorization of a committee is required if the abortion is sought for sociomedical reasons, danger of fetal abnormality, or pregnancy resulting from a sex crime.

Sweden has not yet announced changes in its abortion law, which have been under consideration for three years. Various alternatives are bruited about; that abortion may be permitted on the free choice of the woman provided she consults fully with an abortion service or, possibly, that the decision-making process may be decentralized in order to reduce the current delay which drives many women to illegal abortion.

Abortion on Sociomedical Grounds

Singapore has enacted sociomedical grounds for abortion along the lines of the British Abortion Act of 1967 but with approval required by a Termination of Pregnancy Authorization Board, except when abortion is to preserve life or health(41). This is the first Asian country, after Japan, to enact a liberalized abortion law.

The state of South Australia has also enacted an abortion law modeled after the new British law(42). Similar legislation is under discussion in New South Wales. A poll of general practitioners in Sydney, N.S.W. found that 957 women approached 92 general practitioners with requests for help in obtaining an abortion in a single year(43). The fact that each general practitioner is confronted with a major dilemma of this kind ten times a year explains the high proportion of general practitioners in Sydney (76 percent) who favor liberalization of the law.

Since 1965, the German Democratic Republic has liberalized interpretation of its law, so that abortion is now authorized on sociomedical grounds(44).

Legislation is still pending in India, which in the form proposed would allow abortion on sociomedical grounds and in cases of contraceptive failure(45).

Experience in England, Wales, and Scotland during the first 18 months of the operation of the 1967 British abortion law reveals a shift from illegal to legal abortion, a shift from the private sector to the National Health Service, a slowing down of the illegitimacy rate (47 percent of all abortions in the first 18 months were for single women), and a narrowing of regional discrepancies in the operation of the law(46). With the aid of voluntary pregnancy advisory services, abortion is being made available to women in all geographic areas and income groups(47). Attitudes of gynecologists are becoming more sympathetic to applicants for abortion, as reflected by "the granting of National Health Service abortions on an increasing scale and by bodies such as the Royal College of Obstetricians and Gynaecologists taking a sincere, if belated, interest in contraception and sterilisation"(48). The most serious problem appears to be the universal need for improving contraceptive services and practices.

Abortion on Medical Grounds

Canada(49) and Peru(50) have broadened their abortion laws to permit abortion on the grounds of danger to the life or health of the woman.

Abortion Only to Save the Life of the Woman

This category has lost adherents. It will continue to do so as current law reform activities in many countries, e.g., France, increase in tempo.

INSIGHTS FROM ABROAD

As the United States moves into the problems associated with providing medical care under its new abortion laws, several lessons from the experience of other nations seem relevant.

1. A liberal abortion law will transfer a number of illegal abortions to safe, clinical practice; but as long as restrictions in grounds or procedures remain, some illegal abortion will persist(51). Initial experience under the California Therapeutic Abortion Act confirms this finding(52). Therefore, experience in the four states that have removed virtually all restrictions will be extremely important.

2. The earlier in pregnancy that abortion is provided, the less tendency there is to resort to illegal abortion. In eastern Europe, where abortion is generally done early in pregnancy, illegal abortion has been

almost eliminated. The reverse is true in Sweden, where administrative procedures delay authorization for legal abortion. The U. S. laws specify time periods within which the abortion must be performed, but, in addition, women should be educated to seek abortions early and procedures should be simplified to achieve this objective.

3.   On the basis of experience from eastern Europe, mortality from legal abortion can be anticipated to be low, particularly if performed early in pregnancy(53). Complications in eastern Europe affect less than three percent of patients(54). England, as yet, has insufficient data on morbidity. One British authority has suggested that the requirement of a medical report within seven days after the abortion is too short a time to provide accurate information on complications(55). Accurate records and reporting are essential.

4.   As the British experience indicates, the climbing rate of illegitimacy in the United States may be slowed by increased availability of abortion. With nearly ten percent of all U. S. births in 1967 illegitimate, the option of abortion will need to be made widely known and accessible if the risks to health and the social disabilities of births to unmarried mothers are to be lessened(56).

5.   Uneven application of the law by reason of varying attitudes on the part of physicians can be anticipated from the experience in England and Norway. California's experience is similar. Continuing education programs for the medical profession and reforms in medical education are urgent.

6.   Shortages of medical and auxiliary personnel may impede full implementation of new laws. In England, however, it was found that, if evenly distributed among all gynecologists, the increased number of abortions would not constitute an excessive workload(57). It has been suggested that in the United States the load might be distributed among a larger group of physicians than those specialized in gynecology, if the social policy expressed by the new laws is to be implemented. Residents and interns on all services might be expected to perform abortions. Nurse-midwives might also be trained and utilized to perform early abortions. Such a decision would require amendment of the licensure laws in the three states that now license nurse-midwives and enactment of such licensure laws in other states.

7.   England's experience shows the bottleneck that may result from shortage of facilities. Ambulatory care, as provided in other countries and as now demonstrated in the United States, is a promising

Statutes provide that abortions are permitted f

State	Year	Physician	Hospital	Life	Health	Physical Health	Mental Health	Fetal Deformity	Forcible Rape	Statutory Rape (Age)	Incest	Time Limit (Weeks)	M.D. Approval	Residency
ALABAMA	1951			✓	✓									
ALASKA	1970	✓	✓[1]									*		✓ 30 d
ARIZONA	1865			✓										
ARKANSAS	1969	✓	✓	✓	✓			✓	✓		✓		3C	✓ 4 mo
CALIFORNIA	1967	✓	✓	✓		✓	✓		✓	✓(15)	✓	✓(20)	2-3B[2]	
COLORADO	1967	✓	✓	✓		✓	✓	✓	✓	✓(16)	✓	✓(16)[3]	3B	
CONNECTICUT	1860			✓										
DELAWARE	1969	✓	✓	✓		✓	✓	✓	✓		✓	✓(20)[4]	1C-RA	✓ 4 mos
DIST. OF COL.	1901			✓	✓									
FLORIDA	1868			✓										
GEORGIA	1968	✓	✓	✓	✓			✓	✓	✓(14)			2C 3B	✓
HAWAII	1970	✓	✓									*		✓ 90 dy
IDAHO	1863			✓										
ILLINOIS	1874			✓										
INDIANA	1838			✓										
IOWA	1843			✓										
KANSAS	1969	✓	✓[7]	✓		✓	✓	✓	✓	✓(16)	✓		3C	
KENTUCKY	1910			✓										
LOUISIANA	1914			✓									1C	
MAINE	1840			✓										
MARYLAND	1968	✓	✓	✓		✓	✓	✓	✓			✓(26)[8]	RA	
MASSACHUSETTS	1845			✓[9]	✓[9]									
MICHIGAN	1846			✓										
MINNESOTA	1851			✓										
MISSISSIPPI	1966	✓		✓					✓[10]	✓[10]			2C	
MISSOURI	1835			✓										

C — Consultant; B — Therapeutic Abortion Board; RA — Hospital Review Authority   *Non-Viable Fetu

[1] Abortion must be "performed in a hospital or other facility approved for the purpose by the Department of Health an Welfare or a hospital operated by the federal government or an agency of the federal government . . ." Abortion ma not be performed unless "consent has been received from the parent or guardian of an unmarried woman less than 1 years of age . . ."

[2] Two-member abortion board required through the 12th week of pregnancy, three-member board thereafter.

[3] The 16-week time limit applies to rape and incest only.

[4] After 20 weeks a pregnancy may be terminated to preserve the woman's life or where the fetus is dead.

[5] Residency requirement does not apply if the woman or her husband works in Delaware or if she has previously been patient of a Delaware physician or if her life is in danger.

[6] "The affidavit [re: residency] of such a woman shall be prima facie evidence of compliance with this requirement."

[7] Abortion must be done in a hospital "or other place as may be designated by law . . ."

[8] After 26 weeks a pregnancy may be terminated to preserve maternal life or when the fetus is dead.

Primary sources: *Checklist of Abortion Laws in the United States.* Association for the Study of Abortion, Inc., 1970.
Lader, Lawrence. "A National Guide to Legal Abortion." *Ladies' Home Journal,* July 1970.

Prepared by NATIONAL CENTER FOR FAMILY PLANNING SERVICES, HSMHA, HEW.

ABORTION LAWS - January 1971

e reasons indicated and under the conditions specified.

State	Year	Physi-cian	Hospi-tal	Life	Health	Physi-cal Health	Men-tal Health	Fetal Deform-ity	Forc-ible Rape	Statu-tory Rape (Age)	Incest	Time Limit (Weeks)	M.D. Appro-val	Resi-dency
ONTANA	1864			√										
EBRASKA	1873			√										
EVADA	1861			√										
EW HAMPSHIRE	1848			√										
EW JERSEY	1849			√[11]										
EW MEXICO	1969	√	√	√		√	√	√	√	√(16)	√		2B	
EW YORK	1970	√										√(24)[12]		
CAROLINA	1967	√	√	√	√			√	√		√		3C	√4 mos.
DAKOTA	1943			√										
HIO	1841			√										
KLAHOMA	1910			√										
REGON	1969	√	√	√		√[13]	√[13]	√	√	√(16)	√	√150 dys[14]	1C	√
ENNSYLVANIA[15]	1860													
UERTO RICO	1913			√										
HODE ISLAND	1896			√										
CAROLINA	1970	√	√	√		√	√	√	√		√		3C	√90 days
DAKOTA	1929			√										
ENNESSEE	1883			√										
EXAS	1859			√										
TAH	1876			√										
ERMONT	1867			√										
IRGINIA	1970	√	√	√		√	√	√	√		√		Board	√120 dys[16]
ASHINGTON	1970	√	√[17]									√(16)		√90 days
EST VIRGINIA	1848			√										
ISCONSIN	1858			√									2C	
YOMING	1869			√										

The statute prohibits "unlawful" abortion, or abortion which is "malicious" or performed "without lawful justification." Case law, however, sanctions abortion to preserve maternal life and protect maternal health. COMMONWEALTH V. WHEELER (1944).

Statute does not specify whether forcible or statutory rape (or either) is meant.

The statute forbids abortions done "maliciously or without lawful justification." Case laws provide that abortions are permitted at least to preserve the life of the woman, GLEITMAN V. COSGROVE (1967).

[12] After 24 weeks pregnancy may be terminated only to preserve woman's life.

[13] "In determining whether or not there is substantial risk [to her physical or mental health] account may be taken of the mother's total environment, actual or reasonably foreseeable."

[14] The 150-day time limit does not apply in cases of danger to life.

[15] "Unlawful" abortion is proscribed but not defined.

Residency may be proved by affidavit.

[17] Abortion must be performed in an accredited hospital or medical facility approved by the state Board of Health. Pregnancy can be lawfully terminated "with the prior consent and, if married and residing with her husband or unmarried and under the age of 18 years, with the prior consent of her husband or legal guardian, respectively."

NOTE: Provided in military facilities in the U. S. without regard to local State laws (Dr. L. Rousselot, Deputy Assistant Secretary of Defense for Health and Environment, May 22 & July 31, 1970).

solution for early abortions. Moreover, ambulatory treatment reduces the cost of abortions.

8.   Evidence from Chile, South Korea, and Taiwan indicates that, in a country with a high or increasing abortion rate, the conditions are favorable for effective family planning programs(58). A possible hazard is that the easy solution of abortion may generate a lack of responsibility in using contraceptives. Zeal to meet a long-neglected human need should be accompanied by efforts to use abortion as a means of encouraging effective contraception. A number of European statutes prohibit abortion if an abortion has been performed in the preceding six-month period. A more effective deterrent to repeated abortion would consist in aiding every woman who has an abortion to obtain and use effective methods of contraception.

The dynamic legislative and judicial developments in the laws governing abortion in the United States have generated a groundswell of change. The action of the U. S. Supreme Court is crucial to the rate of progress, but, regardless of the outcome of cases pending before the Court, the clock can never be turned back. Safe, legal abortion is now recognized as a fundamental right of women, a protection of maternal health and family welfare, and an assurance that every child is a loved and wanted child. Abortion, however, should be only one service in an array of services that should also include effective contraception, education for responsible sexual relationships, and health protection for mothers and children.

REFERENCES

1. American Law Institute, Model Penal Code, sec. 230.3(2) (Proposed Official Draft, 1962). On Aug. 4, 1970 the Commissioners on Uniform State Laws issued a Second Tentative Draft of a Uniform Abortion Act, which authorizes abortions within 24 weeks after commencement of the pregnancy without specific grounds or after 24 weeks on the grounds set forth in the Code. The 12 statutes incorporating all or part of the Model Penal Code are: Ark. Stat. Ann., secs. 41-301 to 41-310 (Supp. 1969); Cal. Health & Safety Code Ann., secs 25950-54 (Supp. 1970); Colo. Rev. Stat. Ann., secs. 40-2-50 to 40-2-53 (Supp. 1967); Del. Code Ann., tit. 11, sec. 301 (1953) and Laws 1969; Ga. Code Ann., secs. 26-9920a to 26-9925a (1969); Kan. Stat. Ann., sec. 21-3407 (Supp. 1969) and Laws 1969; Md. Ann. Code, art. 43, secs. 149E to 149G (Supp. 1969); Miss. Code Ann., sec. 2223 (Supp. 1968); N.M. Stat. Ann., secs. 40A-5-1 to 40A-5-3 (Supp. 1969); N.C. Gen. Stat., secs. 14-44 to 14-45.1 (1969 Replacement Vol. 1B); S.C. Code, secs. 16-82 to 86 (1962) and Laws 1970; Va. Code Ann., secs. 18.1-62 to 18.1-62.3 (Supp. 1970). For discussion of these laws, see Lucas, Roy, Laws of the United States in *Abortion in a Changing World* (Robert E. Hall, Editor), vol. I, p. 127, Columbia Univ. Press, 1970.

2. The American College of Obstetricians and Gynecologists has recently liberalized its position further to approve abortion on the decision of the patient and her physician without additional medical consultation. *AMA News*, Sept. 28, 1970.

3. Elizabeth II, Ch. 87 (1967) permitting termination of pregnancy on the opinion of two registered medical practitioners that continuance of the pregnancy would involve risk to the life of the pregnant woman or injury to the physical or mental health of any existing children of her family greater than if the pregnancy were terminated.

4. S.B. 193, amending Ore. Rev. Stat., secs. 465.110, 677.188, and 677.190 and repealing sec. 163.060 (Laws 1969).

5. S.B. No. 527 repealing and re-enacting Alaska Stat., sec. 11.15.060 (Laws 1970).

6. Public Law No. 1 amending Hawaii Rev. Stat., ch. 768 (Laws 1970).

7. N.Y. Penal Law, sec. 125.05(3) (McKinney Supp. 1970-71).

8. Many states require that the hospital be not only licensed but accredited. For discussion of the unreasonableness and probable unconstitutionality of a requirement restricting performance of abortions to hospitals accredited by the Joint Commission on Accreditation of Hospitals, see Brief *Amici Curiae*, Ass'n for the Study of Abortion, Inc., Planned Parenthood Ass'n, et al. in Vuitch v. Maryland, 271 A. 2d 371 (Court of Special Appeals of Maryland, Nov. 24, 1970).

9. International Herald Tribune, p.3, Aug. 19, 1970.

10. Personal communication from Roy Lucas, President and Associate Counsel, The James Madison Constitutional Law Institute, N.Y., Oct. 22, 1970.

11. 71 Cal. 2d 954, 458 P. 2d 194, 80 Cal. Rptr. 354 (1969), cert. denied, 397 U.S. 915 (1970).

12. *Id.* at 963, 458 P. 2d at 199.

13. 305 F. Supp. 1032 (D.D.C. 1969), ques. of juris. postponed to merits, 397 U.S. 1061, further juris. questions propounded, 399 U.S. 923 (1970) (No. 84, Oct. 1970 Term). On the practical availability of abortion under D.C. law, see court order requiring the D.C. General Hospital to give abortions to women meeting the standards for admission to the hospital. Doe v. Gen'l Hosp. of D.C., 313 F. Supp. 1170 (D.D.C. 1970), on motions to hold hospital officials in contempt,_F. 2d_No. 24,011 (D.C. Cir. Mar. 20 & May 15, 1970).

14. Roe v. Wade, 314 F. Supp. 1217 (N.D. Tex. 1970) (per curiam), appeal docketed, 39 U.S.L.W. 3151 (U.S. Oct. 7, 1970) (No. 808, Oct. 1970 Term).

15. McCann v. Babbitz, 306 F. Supp. 400 (E.D. Wis. 1969) (three judge court convened), 310 F. Supp. 293 (1970) (per curiam) (on the merits), appeal dismissed, 400 U.S._, 39 U.S.L.W. 3132 (Oct. 13, 1970) (per curiam), perm. injunction issued,_F. Supp._(E.D. Wis. Nov. 18, 1970) (per curiam).

16. Rosen v. La. State Bd. Med. Examiners, 318 F. Supp. 1217(1970), (Cassibry, J., dissenting).

17. Planned Parenthood Ass'n of Phoenix v. Nelson, Civ. No. 70-334 PHX (D. Ariz. Aug. 24, 1970) (per curiam).

18. Doe v. Scott,_F. Supp._(N.D. Ill. 1971) (Illinois statue held unconstitutional as impermissibly vague and unduly infringing on the woman's right of privacy in restricting abortion during the first trimester of pregnancy by a licensed physician in a licensed facility).

19. YWCA v. Kugler, Civ. No. 264-70 (D.N.J., filed Mar. 5, 1970).

20. Crossen v. Breckenridge, Civ. No. 2143 (E.D. Ky.), dismissed June 15, 1970 by U. S. Judge Swinford, Lexington (Ky.) Herald, June 16, 1970. On appeal.

21. Doe v. Randall, 314 F. Supp. 32 (D. Minn. 1970), rehearing denied, 314 F. Supp. 36 (D. Minn. July 1, 1970) (per curiam), appeal docketed *sub nom.* Hodgson v. Randall, 39 U.S.L.W. 3115 (Sept. 21, 1970) (No. 728, Oct. 1970 Term).

22. Hall v. Lefkowitz, 305 F. Supp. 1030 (S.D.N.Y. 1969), dismissed as moot, Op. No. 36936 (S.D.N.Y. July 1, 1970) (per curiam).

23. People v. Anast, No. 69-3429 (Ill. Cir. Ct., Cook County, 1970) (Dolezal, J.).

24. Commonwealth v. Page, Centre County Leg. J. at 285 (Pa. Ct. Comm. Pl., Centre County July 23, 1970).

25. State v. Munson (S.D. 7th Jud. Cir., Pennington County Apr. 6, 1970) (Clarence P. Cooper, J.).

26. State v. Ketchum (Mich. Dist. Ct. Mar. 30, 1970) (Reid, J.).

27. Kudish v. Bd. of Registration in Med., 355 Mass._, 248 N.E. 2d 264 (1969). Similar decisions have upheld the Iowa and Vermont statues as not unconstitutionally vague.

28. See, for example, Arnold v. Sendak, No. IP 70-C-217 (S.D. Ind., filed Mar. 29, 1970); Rodgers v. Danforth, Civ. No. 18360-2 (W.D. Mo., filed May 15, 1970); Steinberg v. Brown, No. C-70-289 (N.D. Ohio); Doe v. Rampton, Civ. No. 234-70 (D. Utah, Sept. 14, 1970) (Temporary restraining order against enforcement of Utah statue issued).

29. Corkey v. Edwards, Civ. No. 2665 (W.D.N.C., filed May 12, 1970); Gwynne v. Hicks, Civ. No. 70-1088-CC (C.D. Calif., filed May 18, 1970); Doe v. Dunbar, Civ. No. C-2402 (D. Colo., filed July 2, 1970), juris. granted_F. Supp._(D. Colo. Dec. 22, 1970). (One of the attorneys in the Colorado suit challenging the first ALI-style law enacted is Richard D. Lamm, sponsor of the reformed legislation in the Colorado Legislature.)

30. Doe v. Bolton,_F. Supp._, Civ. No. 13676 (N.D. Ga. July 31,

1970) (per curiam), appeal docketed, 39 U.S.L.W. 3227 (U.S. Nov. 17, 1970) (Nos. 971, 973, Oct. Term 1970).

31. People v. Robb, Nos. 149005 & 159061 (Calif. Mun. Ct., Orange County, Jan. 9, 1970) (Mast, J.); People v. Gwynne, No. 173309 (Calif. Mun. Ct., Orange County, June 16, 1970) (Thomson, J.); People v. Gwynne, No. 176601 (Calif. Mun. Ct., Orange County, Aug. 13, 1970) (Schwab, J.).

32. People v. Barksdale, No. 33237C (Calif. Mun. Ct., Alameda County, Mar. 24, 1970) (Foley, J.).

33. *Ibid.*

34. The Jurisdictional Statement filed in the U. S. Supreme Court on Oct. 7, 1970 by Roy Lucas et al. in Roe v. Wade, 314 F. Supp. 1217 (N.D. Tex. 1970) (per curiam), No. 808, Oct. 1970 Term cites the following cases at p. 18, n. 30: Muncie v. Missouri, 398 U.S. 938 (June 1, 1970), denying cert. to 448 S.W. 2d 879 (Mo. 1970); California v. Belous, 397 U.S. 915 (Feb. 24, 1970), denying cert. to 71 Cal. 2d 954, 458 P. 2d 194, 80 Cal. Rptr. 354 (1969); Molinaro v. New Jersey, 396 U.S. 365 (Jan. 19, 1970) (per curiam), dismissing appeal from 54 N.J. 246, 254 A. 2d 792 (1969); Knight v. Louisiana Bd. of Medical Examiners, 395 U.S. 933 (June 2, 1969), denying cert. to 252 La. 889, 214 So. 2d 716 (1968) (per curiam); Morin v. Garra, 395 U.S. 935 (June 2, 1969), denying cert. to 53 N. J. 82 (1968) (per curiam); Moretti v. New Jersey, 393 U.S. 952 (Nov. 18, 1968), denying cert. to 52 N. J. 182, 244 A. 2d 499 (1968); Fulton v. Illinois, 390 U.S. 953 (Mar. 4, 1968), denying cert. to 84 Ill. App. 2d 280, 228 N.E. 2d 203 (1967); Carter v. Florida, 376 U.S. 648 (Mar. 30, 1964), dismissing appeal from 150 So. 2d 787 (Fla. 1963).

35. McCann v. Babbitz, 310 F. Supp. 293 (E.D. Wis. 1970), appeal dismissed, 400 U.S.__, 39 U.S.L.W. 3132 (Oct. 13, 1970) (per curiam), supra note 15.

36. Roemer, R.   Abortion Law: The Approaches of Different Nations, *Am. J. Pub. H.*, vol. *57*, no. 11, p. 1906, Nov. 1967; Roemer, R.   Abortion Laws of the World: Recent Trends and Policy Issues   in *Abortion in a Changing World, supra* note 1 at p. 119.

37. Bulgaria. Law of 16 Feb. 1968, Int. Dig. Health Leg., vol. 19, pp. 589-602, 1968.

38. David, Henry P. *Family Planning and Abortion in the Socialist Countries*

of Central and Eastern Europe, A Compendium of Observations and Readings, p. 69, The Population Council, New York, 1970.

39. Finland. Law No. 239 of 24 Mar. 1970 on the interruption of pregnancy, Int. Dig. Health Leg., vol. 21 no. 4, 1970.

40. Denmark. Law of 18 Mar. 1970, Int. Dig. Health Leg., vol. 21, no. 3, 1970.

41. The Abortion Act of Singapore, 1969, Republic of Singapore, passed 29 Dec. 1969 and assented to by the President 31 Dec. 1969, Int. Dig. Health Leg., vol. 21, no. 4, 1970.

42. South Australia. An Act to amend the Criminal Consolidation Act, 1935-1966, No. 109 of 1969, assented to 8 Jan. 1970.

43. Sussman, William and Anthony I. Adams. General Practitioners' Views on Pregnancy Termination, *Med. J. of Australia,* pp. 169-173, July 25, 1970.

44. *Supra* note 38 at p. 233.

45. India, The Medical Termination of Pregnancy Bill, 1969 (Bill No. XXII of 1969).

46. Diggory, Peter and Malcolm Potts. Preliminary Assessment of the 1967 Abortion Act in Practice, *The Lancet,* pp. 287-291, Feb. 7, 1970.

47. *Id.* at p. 290.

48. *Ibid.*

49. Stats. of Canada, C. 38, sec. 18 (1968-69).

50. Peru. Decree-Law No. 17505 of 18 Mar. 1969, Ch. II, sec. 19, Int. Dig. Health Leg., vol. 21, p. 137 at 140, 1970.

51. Potts, D. Malcolm. Induced Abortion—the Experience of Other Nations in *Population Control, Implications, Trends, and Prospects,* Proceedings of the Pakistan International Family Planning Conference at Dacca, Jan. 28 - Feb. 4, 1969, p. 241, Sweden Pakistan Family Welfare Project, Lahore, West Pakistan, March 1969.

52. See California State Department of Public Health, *A Report to the 1970 Legislature, Third Annual Report on the Implementation of the California Therapeutic Abortion Act,* p. 5 estimating that 81,600 abortions were done on California women in 1968, of which 76,600 were illegal. Even substantially increased numbers of therapeutic abortions—which have occurred since 1968—will not eliminate an illegal abortion problem of this magnitude. The source of the estimated number of illegal abortions was a carefully

controlled study in North Carolina. Abernathy, James R., Bernard G. Greenberg, and Daniel G. Horvitz. Estimates of Induced Abortion in Urban North Carolina, *Demography*, vol. 7, no. 1, p. 19, Feb. 1970.

53. See Tietze, Christopher. Abortion Laws and Practices in Europe, *Excerpta Medica International Congress*, Series No. 207 April 1969 and Tietze, Christopher. Mortality with Contraception and Induced Abortion, *Studies in Family Planning*, vol. 45, p. 6, Sept. 1969.

54. *Supra* note 38 at p. 253.

55. *Supra* note 46 at p. 290.

56. On the higher risks of the unmarried mother and her child, see *Health Aspects of Family Planning*, Report of a WHO Scientific Group, World Health Organization Technical Rept. Series, No. 442, p. 10, Geneva, 1970.

57. *Supra* note 46 at p. 288.

58. Engstrom, Lars Erik. Abortion as a Method of Population Control, in *Population Control, Implications, Trends, and Prospects, Supra* note 51 at p. 240.

Chapter 6

The Destiny of the Unwanted Child: The Issue of Compulsory Pregnancy

Mildred B. Beck

Much has been written about the consequences of unwanted pregnancy for the pregnant woman, the father, and others significantly related to them. Strikingly little, by contrast, has been written—or is known—about the fate of the child compelled to be born against the wishes of his mother, his father, or both. Yet he is, to say the least, an interested party. Ironically, though he has many spokesmen, they do not speak with one voice. Nor do these spokesmen truly represent him, for they are self-designated, express their personal views, and fight for what *they* believe is good for children. When the "good" is described in diametrically conflicting terms, however, it is desirable wherever possible to separate fact from fancy, conjecture from evidence, and wishful thinking from reality.

I address myself here to what is known to be true, even within the limited state of present knowledge, and I will suggest areas of needed research. As a necessary preliminary, I define "compulsory pregnancy"* to mean a particular pregnancy, incurred by chance or by plan, which for any reason whatsoever is steadfastly and unequivocally unwanted by the pregnant woman, but which she is compelled by external circumstances to carry to term. The qualifying words are intended to

---

*I am indebted for this term to Garrett Hardin who, to the best of my knowledge, coined it. Its currency is a mark of its usefulness.

preclude the transitory ambivalence that may have assailed virtually every pregnant woman since the beginning of time.

There are extremely important differences between women who say "I *never* want to become pregnant" and those who say "I do not want *this* pregnancy" for one or more of the following reasons:

1.   I am told that my child, on the basis of medical findings, stands a substantial chance of being severely deformed or retarded. (This includes rubella victims, cases where the fetus is at risk for genetic reasons, cases where the parent has used damaging drugs, etc.).

2.   The doctor warned me against another pregnancy because I have a severe heart condition (or some other life-threatening or life-shortening disability).

3.   I can barely care for the three (four, five, six. . . .) children I already have.

4.   My husband has just returned from Vietnam and he is under an incredible strain that I don't understand. I just can't look after our other kids and him, too . . . and, my God, another baby!

5.   This baby is cursed, just as all my father's other children are(1).

6.   We've practiced birth control effectively until now and our children are spaced just as we wanted them. I don't want this baby; in fact, I just can't raise another.

7.   You aren't going to let her have this kid, are you? She's only twelve herself!

8.   I never really wanted a baby; I just wanted to see if I could get pregnant. I hate kids!

9.   We'll *have* to marry if I am forced to have this baby because my parents insist. But they can have the baby and you can have the father. I won't live with him for a minute!

Highly responsible persons who seek to terminate a pregnancy do so because of concern for the outcome for themselves, the child-to-be, and others close to them whose lives are adversely affected by the unwanted pregnancy. There also are women, characterized by varying degrees of "immaturity." Assuming that society has an interest in reducing uncontrolled, and some forms of uncontrollable, sexual behavior, how can this be done? By compelling a woman to carry to term an unwanted pregnancy, placing in her custody an absolutely helpless and hapless infant? Is there any evidence to suggest that this is a successful method? And what is the cost to the infant? Erik Erikson, in *Childhood and Society*, contends that "the firm establishment of enduring patterns . . . of basic trust . . . is the first task of the ego, and thus the first task for maternal care. But . . . the amount of trust derived from earliest infantile experience [depends] on *the quality of the maternal relationship*. Mothers create a sense of trust in their children. . . . This forms the basis in the child for a sense of identity which will later combine a sense of being 'all right,' or being oneself, and of becoming what other people trust one will become"(2). One must, then, inquire *whose* interests are served by compulsory pregnancy, and into the outcome for each of the principals.

In this presentation, the "unwanted child" is seen as the product of a compulsory (unwanted) pregnancy, whether or not the mother seeks a legal or an illegal abortion, or whether or not she attempts to abort herself. Legal abortions still are for the few who have luck, influential friends, money, or who can borrow substantial sums. Available statistics indicate that each year some 10,000 women have legal abortions; estimates of the incidence of illegal and self-induced abortion range between 200,000 and 1,200,000. In addition, an unknown number of women make unsuccessful attempts at inducing abortion, and in these cases one can only speculate about the damage they may have done to themselves or to the child.

The unwanted child is characterized by one or more of the following:

1.   He has biological parents only. Although he is rarely, often never, seen by his parents after birth, he is not necessarily released for adoption or other long-term care. At times the parent cannot be found, or refuses to become involved in any way in the care of, or planning for, the child or, even when the law permits the legal termination of parenthood, withholds consent. (Agencies sometimes fail to terminate parental rights, even when it is legally permissible, because an adoptive home cannot be found, perhaps because of race, religion, or because the child is physically or mentally handicapped.)

2.   He is abandoned: wrapped in a paper bag or newspaper, and left in a refuse can; or perhaps left, unfed, and sometimes injured, on a doorstep, or in a hallway, or with a "sitter," often a person relatively unknown to the parents.

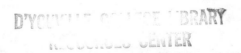

3.   He is neglected or abused in the sense that, if the child were brought to the attention of the courts, there would ensue a legal finding of neglect or abuse. Here we include children suffering from severe malnutrition although the mother does not lack knowledge of nutrition, and there is no evidence of financial need; the infant or young child who is left for days on end with some vague provision for someone to look in on him from time to time; the children left for prolonged periods in so-called well-baby wards of hospitals, or in shelters, or in emergency foster care when there is no demonstrable evidence of need or when the mother offers one excuse after another for failing to provide for the child in any way whatsoever.

Such are the circumstances of the lives of unwanted children. A few details complete this unhappy picture. Many of the mothers of these children have tried to get contraceptive help, and later an abortion, but to no avail. Many of these women are mentally and emotionally ill or retarded. Some are drug addicts or alcoholics. With shocking frequency, they were, more often than not, themselves the object of childhood abuse. Another group, of unknown size, present a curious phenomenon. Dr. Gerald Caplan of the Harvard School of Public Health found that young children were brought to a child guidance clinic by mothers who—except in their relationship to the patient—were warm, generous, good mothers. During the course of treatment almost every mother "confessed" that she tried to abort the patient, and—considering the nature of these efforts—she was sure the child was damaged. She responds to the child as though it had actually been impaired by her; furthermore, she comes to believe that the child knows what she "tried to do to him," and she then ascribes to the child a deliberate talent for meanness and revenge in his response to her. What a tragic penalty must be paid by the unwitting victim! Clearly, where unwanted children are concerned, we must ask not only who punishes whom, but also how much society itself is *compelled* to pay for the human suffering that it unintentionally imposes.

Lacking definitive studies of the outcome, over periods of time, of compulsory pregnancies, contending factions are in a position to defend cherished theories. It is possible, for example, that a child born of a compulsory pregnancy may become the most loved and treasured of children. And a few of these children may indeed become Beethovens or Michelangelos. But how many of these potential geniuses disappear into anaclitic depressions after spending months in institutional well-baby wards? And how many lesser lights are dimmed or extinguished by neglect? In fact, many thousands of babies and young children become unplaceable *after* society has intervened in their behalf because suitable foster and adoptive homes are not available to them until months or years after they are first needed.

HISTORICAL PERSPECTIVE

A few statistics may be illuminating. According to Dr. Robert Hall, abortion before "quickening" was not proscribed by religious groups in the western world until 1803. The first anti-abortion law in the United States was not passed until 1835. And it was not until 1869 that, for the first time, early abortion was viewed as murder by the Catholic Church.

Until 1966, forty-five American states defined abortion as unlawful unless it was necessary to preserve the *life* and, in five states and the District of Columbia, the *health* of the mother. Interestingly, the abortion rate was the same in all states, despite the more liberal interpretation in the latter five states, probably because competent and concerned physicians everywhere have often elected to protect the *health* of the woman irrespective of the law. But concern for the welfare of the infant, despite such known hazards as rubella and certain genetic disorders, was not an indication for abortion in any state. Yet long before 1966 physicians aborted women for these and other reasons in keeping with the dictates of their professional and ethical beliefs and their deep concern for human welfare. Still, in most states today, conscientious and law-abiding physicians must continue to make the terrible choice between permitting virtually inevitable tragedy or of skirting the law and practicing medicine that is in accord with modern medical knowledge.

We should remember that public relations and promotional techniques were not invented by Madison Avenue. Our predecessors had some effective techniques of their own. They elicited—only too successfully—the offices of the church and related institutions, reinforcing all with the power of the law. The problem today is: How do we reform or repeal laws that have fulfilled their mission, and proceed to take account of new knowledge, accumulated experience, and contemporary values?

At the moment we often find ourselves in untenable positions. For instance, it is extremely difficult to demonstrate that a woman is at risk, physicially or mentally, as some of the liberalized abortion laws demand. Certifying that a pregnant woman's life or health is at risk "temporarily or with medical certainty" as a direct consequence of the pregnancy asks physicians and psychiatrists to be clairvoyant. Yet, the danger to the physical and mental well-being of the mother and child is far greater, certainly over time, than the law recognizes. Worst of all, the laws are applied capriciously, inequitably and—not infrequently—hypocritically. Here attention is called to the testimony of those who serve on, or are associated with, hospital abortion committees. As for the discriminatory application of the law, Robert Hall has reported that "private patients get hospital abortions four times as often as ward patients"(3).

Unwanted children have been born throughout recorded history, but they have been dealt with differently from one period to another. It should be remembered that the Society for the Prevention of Cruelty to *Animals* first appeared in England in 1824, and in the United States in 1866. The Society for the Prevention of Cruelty to *Children* was established in the United States five years later. This is only one of countless indications throughout recorded history illustrating, not that we care more about animals than children, but that most human beings cannot bring themselves to reflect upon the depth and the extent of the suffering of children.

In the past unwanted children were dealt with much more forthrightly though not always more inhumanely than today. Infanticide, *by contrast* not the worst fate that can befall an infant, is described from earliest times. As recently as the eighteenth and nineteenth centuries, overt as well as disguised infanticide was commonplace. William Langer, discussing conditions in Europe, makes this plain:

In the cities it was common practice to confide babies to old woman nurses or caretakers. The least offense of the "Angelmakers," as they were called . . . , was to give children gin to keep them quiet. [According to Disraeli], "Laudanum and treacle, administered in the shape of some popular elixir, affords these innocents a brief taste of the sweets of existence and, keeping them quiet, prepares them for the silence of their impending grave. . . . Infanticide is practiced as extensively and as legally in England as it is on the banks of the Ganges. . . .

The middle and late 18th Century was marked by a startling rise in the rate of illegitimacy [and] so many of the unwanted babies were being abandoned, smothered or otherwise disposed of that Napoleon in 1811 decreed that foundling hospitals should be provided with a turntable device, so that babies could be left at these institutions without the parent being recognized or subjected to embarrassing questions. This convenient arrangement was imitated in many countries and was taken full advantage of. . . . Of the thousands of children thus abandoned, more than half were the offspring of married couples. . . .

Most of the children died within a short time, either of malnutrition or neglect. . . . In some of the Italian hospitals the mortality ran to 80 or 90 percent. In Paris the Maison de la Couche reported that of 4,779 babies admitted in 1818, 2,370 died in the first three months and another 956 within the first year. . . . Many contemporaries denounced [this system] as legalized infanticide, and one . . . suggested that the foundling hospitals post a sign reading, "Children killed at Government expense."

In light of the available data one is almost forced to admit that the proposal, seriously advanced at the time, that unwanted babies be painlessly asphyxiated in small gas chambers was definitely humanitarian(4).

How do unwanted children fare today? Are we asking the right questions, the basic questions as to *why* we have so many? Have we investigated the fate of these children from the moment the *unwanting mother* perceives that she is pregnant? And what responsibility do those who staunchly fight for the rights of the fetus assume, *postnatally*, to ensure the fulfillment of these rights? Finally, since society dictates most of the conditions under which we live, what does society do for the unwanted child?

We may never get accurate figures on the number of unplanned and unwanted pregnancies and children in the United States, but we have clues. According to Dr. Alan Guttmacher, President of Planned

Parenthood/World Population, four out of five American couples practice some form of birth control after a first child is born but, because of contraceptive failure due to unreliability of the method or careless use, about half of their subsequent pregnancies are unplanned(5). And in 1967, 318,000, or slightly more than 9 percent of all United States births were illegitimate, and approximately 40 percent of these births were to mothers 15-19 years of age(6). In all probability the recorded number of illegitimate births would be substantially increased were it not for false birth certificates. Add babies born to couples whose marriages were enforced by parental or other pressures, and the presumed number of unwanted infants rises sharply(7).

If it were true, as some assert, that the unwanted infant usually becomes wanted after birth, why are so many babies and young children abandoned? Why are more than 300,000 American children, according to Child Welfare League and U.S. Children's Bureau estimates, in foster care on any given day? How does it happen that 100,000 of these children are trapped in foster care and have virtually no hope of returning to their own homes—if ever there was one? And how can we explain the 46 percent of the children currently in foster care who are there because of "parental neglect, abuse, or exploitation?" As for the others, broken homes, economic problems, disabling physical and mental disabilities of one or both parents characterize nearly all as "orphans of the living."

If prenatal care is of value in ensuring a healthy mother and infant, its absence is a loss. But how many women, bent on getting an abortion, are likely to seek prenatal care or to avail themselves of it even when it is offered? We have evidence that an unwanted pregnancy sets a destructive process in motion. One need only talk with unwillingly pregnant women—married or unmarried, too young to be a "teenager" or old enough to be menopausal, rich or poor, of any skin hue. Hear them describe what they have tried in order to induce abortion; what they will yet do if worse comes to worst; and note their despair, rage, and their sense of utter defeat. The methods that have been employed by desperate women are documented in Norman Himes's classic *Medical History of Contraception*(8). We merely report here that some of these methods are almost beyond the reader's capacity to bear.

Many women, despite incredibly savage and damaging efforts to induce an abortion, fail and come to term. If, as some contend, it is the pregnant woman and not the fetus that suffers prenatal deprivations of all kinds, what kind of mother—physically and psychologically—will she be to that completely dependent and helpless infant? Conversely, if the fetus is susceptible to damage and shock, what degree of permanent harm will have been done to him? As long as we continue to deny abortions to women who want them, we have an obligation to ascertain the fetus's chance of successful survival of the pregnancy as well as the days and months that follow. The defenders of the premise that a child has a right to a decent life of dignity and fulfillment are, in my judgment, obligated to ensure that these conditions are met. Otherwise, the fetus's defenders may condemn him, postnatally, to neglect, abuse, lifelong institutionalization, or the threat of infanticide.

We have long deplored the paucity of data on the outcome of unwanted pregnancy. The allegation that it is impossible to study the outcome of unwanted pregnancies and denied abortions is subject to serious challenge.

If one recalls Victor Hugo's observation that "nothing is as powerful as an idea whose time has come," one will not be surprised that recently a substantial number of articles, studies and unpublished manuscripts have been addressed to the fate of the unwanted child(9). Some of these documents first appeared in obscure scientific or small-audience journals because of the controversial nature of the subject.

On the matter of studying the outcome of denied abortions, the opportunities now only wait to be grasped. As an example, in Maryland there are far more legitimate requests for abortion than current resources can handle, and the growing number of pleas for these services from outside the state must, of necessity, be denied. Why not follow up these women in their home states to ascertain what happens where abortion has been denied? Why not look into the outcome for the hundreds of school-age youngsters who remain in school but who are compelled to come to term with unwanted pregnancies? Further, why not attempt to ascertain what has happened to a woman, known to be pregnant, who suddenly no longer is? Can all these noncompleted pregnancies be subsumed under the rubric of spontaneous abortion? Or did all these women go out of town, deliver their babies in secret, and leave them for an unknown person or agency to care for? What is in store for the babies whose unwanted lives we succeed in saving? Oughtn't we to know? Can we justify not knowing? The staggering cost in money, in alarmingly depleted resources for good foster and adoptive homes and for acceptable group care programs is a stiff penalty not only for the woman who has been forced to bear a child against her will or best judgment, but also for the child. Another highly important researchable area pertains to child abuse, a problem of international concern. All fifty American states have passed laws providing for mandatory reporting of presumed instances of child abuse, and the reporting agents—usually physicians, hospitals, and child care institutions—are assured protection against libel suits. The fact that these laws are not producing the hoped-for results suggests the need for prompt study and appropriate action. We should remember that since the majority of abusive parents have been the victims of abuse in their own youth, it follows that victimized children in their turn may become victimizing adults.

According to Drs. Helfer and Kempe, in the United States in 1967 "tens of thousands of children were severely battered or killed"(10). Dr. David Gil, of Brandeis University, notes that reported rates of child abuse represent "an unknown fraction of actual incidence rates"(10). This under-reporting, according to Katherine B. Oettinger, is due in part to the fact that "there are few topics in modern life that are more repugnant . . . than the abuse of a child by the very persons entrusted with his care. Yet the fact is that some people of every socioeconomic, educational, religious, and geographical background in our society continue to abuse their children." Further, even in states like New York, where legislation provides for mandatory reporting of suspected cases of child abuse, under-reporting is said to be due to the alarming contention that "hospitals and doctors have begun to say there is nothing to be gained by reporting these tragedies. Society doesn't seem ready to do anything about them anyway"(11).

The Battered Child is not an easy book to read. But to cite a few more findings, Drs. Steele and Pollack studied sixty families intensively where significant abuse of infants and small children under the age of three had occurred(12). (Murder is not included in this sample because the authors hold that "direct murder of children is an entirely different phenomenon and is instigated during a single, impulsive act by people who are clearly psychotic.") The parents included:

> laborers, farmers, blue-collar workers, white-collar workers and top professional people. Some were in poverty, some were relatively wealthy, but most were in-between. . . . Educational

achievement ranged from partial grade school to advanced post-graduate degrees. . . . Intellectual ability ranged from IQs in the 70's to superior ratings of 130. . . . The parents ranged from 18 to 40 years of age, the great majority being in the twenties. . . . The great majority were in relatively stable marriages. . . . Religious affiliations included Catholic, Jewish and Protestant. . . . Most families were Anglo-Saxon Americans. . . . True alcoholism was not a problem except in one family and many were total abstainers. . . . The actual attack on the infant is usually made by one parent. . . . The mother was the attacker in fifty instances, the father in seven, in one family both parents attacked and in two instances, it was difficult to determine which parent was primarily involved.

The parents, on psychiatric examination, were found to be suffering from "hysteria, hysterical psychosis, obsessive-compulsive neurosis, anxiety states, depression, schizoid personality traits, schizophrenia, character neurosis and so on" (p. 108).

There are, of course, many complex factors that contribute to child abuse. But few investigators make a systematic attempt to discover how many of the abusive parents had given clues that the pregnancy was unwanted. In fact, many parents feared the pregnancy because they sensed their uncontrollable aggression toward the coming child. For example, "a pre-maritally conceived pregnancy or one which comes too soon after the birth of a previous child . . . may be perceived as public reminders of sexual transgression or as extra, unwanted burdens" (p. 129).

Radbill, in "A History of Child Abuse and Infanticide," (p. 3) traces the maltreatment of children from earliest times. Infanticide has been practiced for population control, the control of family size, because the child was illegitimate, for economic reasons, because of the mother's "illness, death, youth, debauchery, or demands made upon her by the needs of older siblings, . . . or because of the taboo which kept the mother away from the embraces of her husband during the lactation period, or [the superstitious fear] that twins, monstrous births or congenital defects frequently bode evil. . . . During the period of the Caesars, infanticide, always legal in Rome, received the approbation of philosophers like Seneca"(13).

Abuse of children is tragic. But it could be reduced by eliminating compulsory pregnancy, and by helping people to conceive, bear, and cherish children who are wanted and welcomed.

In conclusion I would like to cite a viewpoint of special importance in a democracy, as expressed by R. E. L. Masters:

> Those of us who claim to be reasonable men and women, who are dedicated to bringing about a maximum application of reason to the regulation of human conduct, must not hesitate when it is necessary to collide with the defenders of prohibitions, even in those areas where they are passionate and fanatical to a dangerous and sometimes pathological degree.

> In the nuclear age it is more essential than ever that superstition and ignorance be overcome. The blind emotivity of fanaticism has become too menacing to be tolerable. The irrational, where discernible in moral codes and political systems, must be firmly weeded out. The time for taboo has passed. In the modern world, freedom is to be tampered with only when society's requirements are both reasonable and compelling; and then to the slightest degree possible. The soundest and most urgent of motives must underlie any attempt to tell men and women how to behave and how not to behave. When the forces of totalitarianism are so powerful, the correct choice is to attempt to *expand* the areas of liberty.

> The compelling reasons advanced for prohibitions must have contemporary, not antique, validity. Appeals to various of humanity's gods, prophets, and religions will not do. Having rejected magic and superstition generally, we may scarcely with intelligence and integrity continue to cling to prohibitions transparently magical and superstitious in origin, unless those prohibitions may now be otherwise and adequately justified. For those who wish to base their conduct upon the revelations and edicts of this god or that one, there is the ever-available concept of sin; but only in a theocracy should what is sinful be also necessarily criminal(14).

REFERENCES

1. In *Child Victims of Incest*, the American Humane Association has estimated an incidence of 832,000 cases of incest in the United States in a fifteen-year period.
2. New York: W. W. Norton (2nd edition. Rev. 1963). p. 249. Emphasis added. With the permission of the publisher.
3. *Saturday Review* (7 December 1968), p. 79.
4. Disguised Infanticide. *American Historical Review 69* (1963).
5. The Tragedy of the Unwanted Child. *Parents' Magazine* (June 1964).
6. U. S. Department of Health, Education, and Welfare. *Trends in Illegitimacy: United States 1940-1965* (February 1968), p. 5. [California and New York, first and second in population size, are two of sixteen states which do not record the legitimacy status of the child on birth certificates. Ed.]
7. Please note that Dr. Charles F. Westoff in an address to the annual meeting of Planned Parenthood—World Population on 28 October 1969, "Extent of Unwanted Fertility in the United States," estimated the number of unwanted children born in the United States to be 800,000 per annum.
8. New York: Gamut Press (1963).
9. See the article by Forssman and Thuwe in the appendix. Ed.
10. Incidence of Child Abuse and Demographic Characteristics of Persons Involved. Chapter 2 in Helfer and Kempe (eds.), *The Battered Child*. Chicago: University of Chicago Press (1968). With the permission of the authors.
11. Private communication to the writer from a distinguished New York philanthropist, long associated with the child care field.
12. A Psychiatric Study of Parents Who Abused Infants and Small Children. p. 103 in Helfer and Kempe.
13. Helfer and Kempe, p. 3.
14. R. E. L. Masters. *Patterns of Incest*. The Julian Press (1963).

Chapter 7

Unwanted Children: Four Case Studies

Sally Provence

I have great respect for the adaptability and resiliency of children. The stresses and traumata that they can somehow survive and surmount, or at least master enough to permit a reasonably adequate life adjustment and adaptation to society, compel respect and allow a measured optimism. Nevertheless, I am alarmed at the severe and often irreparable damage suffered by too many children. I believe that it is important for us to seek answers to the question of how to give each child the best possible opportunity to realize the potential with which he is born; and I devote myself daily to this question. Each working day confronts me with real problems in the lives of children, their parents, and other caretakers.

Child rearing is not an easy task, and even the most talented parents, with children well equipped to survive and develop, do not proceed along the path our wishful fantasies might envision. Crises—internal and external—impinge upon us all, as we struggle to survive and prosper in our complex and demanding society.

I now describe four children—unwanted children of unwanted pregnancies—known to me and my colleagues at the Yale Child Study Center. They are not rare and isolated cases; they are typical of thousands of children who are damaged in their early years by flagrant deficits in the experiences that support development. Some are crippled for the rest of their lives, and will transmit their psychosocial pathology to succeeding generations.

Tommy, age seven, is in a residential treatment center for emotionally disturbed children after passing through five foster homes. I first saw him when he was three. He had been admitted to our hospital because of malnutrition and delayed physical and mental development. The story we heard is not uncommon. He was the fourth child born within five years to an immature woman of twenty-two. At the time of his hospitalization, she told us how unhappy she had felt about this, her fourth pregnancy; that having one more child was just too much for her. Childlike, and in precarious physical health, she was unable to cope with the many responsibilities of caring for four young children, and her burden was increased by an alcoholic husband who worked only intermittently. Although he was interested in her and the children at times, he was frequently neglectful or abusive.

Tommy improved during hospitalization and his parents asked for foster care for him. Tragically, no placement could be sustained for very long—twice because of illness of the foster mother; twice because foster parents, at first motivated to help him, became exhausted with his difficult behavior and his limited responsiveness to their efforts. The residential treatment staff will work with Tommy, trying to rehabilitate him so that he can adjust to family life—an objective of great importance in giving him some hope for the future. Physically, he is now in good condition. Intellectually, he functions at a dull normal level. In his ability to learn, to establish controls over his behavior, and to love others, he is crippled. Experience with similar cases has shown that the chances that he will become an adult who can maintain himself and assume appropriate adult responsibilities are not favorable.

Laurie, four years old, was brought to our clinic at sixteen months by her well-to-do parents who feared she was mentally defective. Two older siblings were doing well. In her first year, Laurie had had two caretakers besides the mother, each of whom was devoted to her for a short time. Laurie's mother was a competent, articulate, conscientious person, who devoted much time and effort to community activities and to her two older children. The father was a responsible man, a hardworking partner in a successful business, and devoted to his wife and the two older children.

Laurie, we found, was an unwanted child of an unwanted pregnancy—a pregnancy during which her mother felt unloved and unlovely. She endured the pregnancy as a sentence to be served before she could again return to the world. In Laurie's infancy her mother was unable to feel close to her, to nurture her in the ways that are crucial to an infant's development. She dressed her in beautiful clothing, but gave little of herself. While she was concerned and guilty, she put other things first. The child had no biological defect; her intellectual, emotional, and motor development were delayed and distorted by the deficits in her care. With casework assistance, the parents have been able to modify some of their behavior so that Laurie is more a part of the family and more time is devoted to her. The parents have provided her with a good nursery school and other social and educational experiences. They have made a conscientious effort to understand her needs. Laurie no longer looks like a mentally retarded child, but her learning is erratic and her interactions with others lack richness and depth. She is attached to her parents and siblings, but not closely. Emotionally starved and isolated by intelligent parents in the midst of economic affluence, she is, sadly, a four-year-old shadow of a person. I fear she can be expected to be an inadequate mother to her own children twenty years from now.

Recently our staff was discussing how we might help a teenage married couple and their three-week-old baby girl. The father, who had grown up in an emotionally impoverished and turbulent home and who had been brought up on delinquency charges on several occasions, wishes not so much to be a parent as to have a wife who can provide him with some of what he has missed. His eighteen-year-old wife, who at times feels a strong wish to mother him and to rescue him from his wild ways, was not at all ready to have a baby. She says, "I'm too young to have a baby," and "I want to be able to go out to the movies and have a good time with my husband and friends." She has no relatives on whom she can call for assistance in child rearing. The baby, now a healthy, robust infant of three weeks is "at risk." There are several possibilities open to us in trying to assist the parents: we will, first of all, help them discuss and decide whether they wish to keep the baby at all, a question they have raised but not resolved. Should they decide to keep her, there are possibilities of our mobilizing services that will enable others to share the care of the infant with the parents. Both the mother and the father are impulsive; they fly into rages and often fight with one another. We fear that they will not be able to control themselves when the baby cries or does other things that might anger them. We hope that they can be helped to arrange at least a reasonably favorable life for the child, either through changes in their behavior and attitudes, or by giving up the child for adoption. But there could have been another option for them. Both have expressed the strong feeling that they did not want a baby; they wanted an abortion. Why not?

Charles, the three-year-old second son of an intelligent professional man and his professionally trained wife, was seen in our clinic because the father was deeply concerned about his wife's rejection and beating of the child. Her care of the child, by no means all negative, is nevertheless characterized by unreasonable expectations, anger, and—at times—neglect, which confuse and upset the child and interfere in very significant ways with his learning and general personality development. Study over a period of time revealed that the wife had not wanted the pregnancy, primarily because it occurred at about the time she learned of her husband's affair with another woman. She sought abortion on psychiatric grounds, but her request was denied. There is reason to believe she might have been better able to accept a girl, but the child—born unwanted—had the additional misfortune of being a boy. She viewed him, from the beginning, as a bad and difficult child whose main purpose in life was to bedevil her. Moreover he was used as a pawn in the frequent quarrels between husband and wife. The mother has never expressed any need for change in her own attitudes, and asked that someone change *the child*, so that she can bear to live with him. As in one of the cases above, this couples' pride will not permit them to give the child into the care of others, but they have been unable to change their behavior in ways that would help the child. Do not misunderstand me—they are not "evil" parents; they are *troubled* parents whose own problems make it impossible for them to provide the child with good care. But the damaging impact of their behavior upon the child's development is unmistakable, and our social customs and legal system allow them to continue.

My point is that the harassed, ill, and immature mother of four; the parents who had completed their family and did not want another child; the adolescent couple aware that they were unready for parenthood; and the wife who was impregnated by a husband unfaithful to her—all wanted to terminate the pregnancies, and would have obtained abortions had they been available to them.

My thesis is simple: I am convinced, on the basis of years of clinical experience with many problems of development in childhood, that there are large numbers of unwanted children, the products of unwanted pregnancies. I am convinced that there is a crucially important need to make abortion available, abortion based upon knowledge of human needs and behavior, and free of punitive elements.

Chapter **8**

Informed
Consent
for
Parenthood

E. James Lieberman

Child rearing is the most difficult and important task that most
ordinary mortals will ever undertake. It is the first priority of this and
every nation; costly to do well, and costlier to neglect. We are not doing
a good enough job. We can do better, but the challenge is sobering.

Unwanted pregnancies result in handicapped children. This is a
truism, if one accepts the premise that being unwanted is a
psychological handicap: the newborn baby leaves life's starting gate
with a substantial drag on its tiny ego. Some infants may do quite well
in spite of this handicap; others clearly not. Strange that so little
research has considered wantedness as a factor in life outcomes!

The usual focus on physical handicaps is easier to document.
Pasamanick provides the useful concept, "continuum of reproductive
casualty," ranging from infant death through severe brain damage and
mental retardation to minor learning or behavioral problems manifest
years later(1). Infant mortality is shockingly high in this country,
especially among the poor, the same population which is more likely to
suffer the nonlethal casualties. It might appear that steps taken to
reduce infant mortality would also reduce the other casualties, but this
is not automatically true; it depends upon what steps are taken.
Modern medical technology can save pregnancies that would have been
aborted, or infants that would otherwise have died. Since some of these
children have irreversible brain damage and other serious problems, we
find that as infant mortality is reduced some forms of morbidity
increase.

One plausible and humane way to reduce the incidence of reproductive casualty is to permit people to become parents *only with their own informed consent.* Informed consent for parenthood—analogous to that needed for medical procedures and experiments—means that couples be told whatever is known about their chances to produce and rear a healthy child. They should have access to information about genetics, nutrition, prenatal care, and child rearing. Obviously, such information must begin in high school or before.

Since a wanted pregnancy is much more likely to be a protected one in which "the advantages of modern medical science can become available to all potential and prospective parents before conception, so ensuring that the child shall inherit its birthright of health," the founders of the Peckham Experiment "were convinced that it mattered that parents should be free from sickness before the child was conceived and carried; certain that the parents should want the child, and that they should be able and eager to rear it(2)."

Prenatal care is often too little and too late. Most women do not arrive at the doctor's office until late in the first trimester; by then the fetus may have sustained irreversible damage (from drugs, infection, radiation) of which the woman is unaware. Women inadvertently and unwillingly pregnant are less likely to seek prenatal care. Many will wish for a spontaneous abortion; some will try to induce an abortion. Trying to bring good prenatal care to unhappily pregnant women is like offering food to someone with anorexia. The effort would be better expended in the preconception period. And, for those women who desire it, abortion must be among the medically approved alternatives—for the wellbeing of the patient and her family, present or future. Prenatal care may at times save fetal tissues but not human life; or it may save human life only to sacrifice it to neglect, abuse, or early death.

Edward Collins, a Howard University medical student, put it this way: "Some pregnancies are benign, some are malignant." Unwanted pregnancy is one malignant tumor about which the medical profession is too nervous to be really helpful. Unwanted pregnancy is psychosocially malignant, and obstetric and pediatric complications abound. Physicians have no better way to make the differential diagnosis than to ask the patient. This is what teachers of medicine mean when they urge medical students to consider the whole person. Unfortunately, medicine still weighs the physical much more than the non-physical components of health, and this may account for our poor record in some areas. We physicians find ourselves much more concerned about the long-range effects of pills (or abortion) designed to prevent unwanted pregnancy than we are about the long-range effects of pregnancy(3)!

Perhaps the benign-malignant dichotomy is too gross. It is indelicate to assign to one fetus the connotation "weed," and "flower" to another. Suppose they are all flowers. The wise gardener will even pluck out flowers, perhaps with a pang of sorrow, when they come up too numerous to thrive, too close together. Spacing, timing, and number are surely no less important in the cultivation of budding human beings.

The Prevention of Handicaps: A Doctor's Dilemma

Preventive medicine is difficult to dramatize. There is excitement in the transplantation of a heart, but the prevention of smallpox or polio is dramatic only to those who know something about these dread diseases, and to those who are specifically interested in health statistics. Our reluctance to emphasize the idea of prevention in discussions of handicapped children rests in part on our distaste for appearing insensitive or pessimistic to the handicapped or their parents. Certainly we want to prevent deafness, blindness, and heart disease. Vaccination against rubella, or abortion in case of maternal rubella, serve as prevention. But many handicapped persons are indisputably glad to be alive, including some disabled by the consequences of maternal rubella.

One way to deal with this dilemma is to make every pregnancy, and every child, a wanted one. If the product of a wanted pregnancy is a retarded or crippled or blind child, then the resources of the community must be such that the parents can fulfill their desire to raise the child in the best possible circumstances, discovering for themselves and reminding their neighbors that there are human values—including personality—that do not depend upon "normality" or conventional success.

But in these difficult times we can only expect parents to meet the challenges of normal or exceptional parenthood if they become parents willingly. And until our society does a good deal more for the handicapped children now alive, it is too much to ask women to carry their pregnancies to term unmindful of possible or probable fetal damage.

If society wishes parents to fully accept the challenge of rearing children well, then let the community make better provision for those who cannot compete on an equal basis for the goods of society. In the meantime, the prevention of unwanted pregnancy, including abortion when necessary, is more than mere prevention. It is an enhancement of life, and it supports the right of every child to be reared by someone who cares.

JUDGMENT TAKES A BACK SEAT: COMPULSORY PREGNANCY

Parenthood is too often initiated by falling into a biopsychosocial trap. Society, instead of permitting (much less encouraging) reflection, frustrates the considered judgment of many women about their own readiness for parenthood. It is certainly true that many pregnancies reflect poor judgment: a premature or inappropriate sexual relationship, a contraceptive left in the dresser drawer, an impulsive decision which—on reflection—seems wrong. But when the pregnant woman, reflecting on her situation, decides against having a child, our laws say: "You should have thought of that before. You must accept a child as the penalty for poor judgment. It is too late to exercise good judgment now." This derives from old prejudices toward sex, and takes no account of the wellbeing of children and families.

One factor in the opposition to abortion is, perhaps, the fear that a large number of nice, average, well-adjusted, responsible American women are against motherhood—at least at times—while favoring sex (on their own terms). That sex, in all its complexity and impulsiveness, is directly linked with parenthood, with all its complexity, mundane demands and nonsexual but supreme rewards, this is a physical miracle transformed into a psychological paradox. In this day and age most conjugal sex will take place without the intention to conceive; parenthood will be achieved by deliberate premeditation for more and more couples; and the relationship between sex and reproduction, while still important psychologically, romantically, and poetically, will no longer be very important biologically.

Abortion will be with us until contraception is automatic. Even then there will still be abortion, because some couples will be ambivalent about parenthood. Or they will want to know if they are fertile, and when the question is answered affirmatively, they will be aghast at the consequences. Since no one can know for certain about his or her capacity to reproduce until it has been tested, it is likely that some will always test, even at great cost to themselves.

If the physician does not turn away from the comprehensive needs of his patient, he must surely ask each woman how she feels about being pregnant. Of course, not every pregnant woman "knows," or can permit herself to say, what she *really* feels; there may never have been a pregnant woman who didn't feel *some* ambivalence about her condition. But the physician who assumes that childbirth will inevitably bring out the good old maternal instinct is a superficial observer of the human condition. More likely, he is a slave to his own masculine-cultural biases, viz., if women could stop pregnancies at will, the human race would end; or, pregnancy and childbirth are the fitting and proper consequences of (punishment for) sexual activity; or, it is not important what happens to a child on earth—it must be allowed to live so that it may enter heaven when it dies.

I have encountered each of these views, and others. One medical student opposed abortion-on-request because he feared it would be the end of the human race. When his fellow students pointed out that women, if determined to end the race, could refrain from sexual intercourse, he replied that this was less of a threat—because men could always resort to forcible sex or artificial insemination! This extreme example points to something more general: many persons—and among them even some women—see women as more or less reluctant, but serviceable, breeding boxes for the benefit of mankind. Clearly, those with such a dim view of women should not have much to do with important decisions about pregnancy and motherhood.

Turning to those who fear that promiscuity will take over society if pregnancy can be cancelled at will, let us consider the theory of deterrence. We wish to deter premarital or incautious sex. Do we know any more effective deterrent than punishment? Punishment in the form of unwanted pregnancy has been applied millions of times. It is very well known as a consequence; yet people go on punishing themselves—and the hapless children as well. Modern psychology informs us that the way to shape behavior is to reward desirable behavior and to stop rewarding undesirable behavior. But society continues to reward the kind of behavior that culminates in pregnancy. While there may be some who, knowing abortion was readily available, would indulge in sex when they would otherwise refrain, we should prefer that risk to the certainty of ruining lives by relying on a deterrent that fails so often and so miserably. Since abortion is no picnic, it has a self-contained deterrent. But as a last resort method of birth control it is necessary at times.

Finally, the argument about getting into heaven. No one has a right to impose his religious views on anyone else, although we must be concerned about the morality of an issue. My present moral position is that anything that increases the suffering of children is immoral, even if legal; and conversely, anything which prevents or diminishes the suffering of children cannot be immoral, even if illegal. The owner of the womb has the right to decide whether it shall bear fruit. No child should be compelled to enter the lives of unwilling parents, much less the corridors of understaffed, overcrowded institutions.

Among the numerous and subtle public health issues surrounding abortion, Christopher Tietze of the Population Council has pointed out that social resistance to abortion forces us into a "pharmaceutical blind alley." Because abortion is not readily available, oral contraceptives have to be potent enough to provide 99 percent effectiveness. The large doses of hormones required for such high effectiveness account for many side effects, including fatal ones. If 90 percent effectiveness were sufficient, with abortion available for contraceptive failures, miniscule doses would suffice, and the pharmacologic risk to millions of women would be greatly reduced.

Psychiatrists and other third parties should not be called upon to decide for or against an abortion. They should be willing to consult when the woman or her physician requests it, but not otherwise(4). "Mental health" grounds for abortion are humane but vague; there is no better judge of the question than the pregnant woman. In any case, since there are too few psychiatrists to handle all the cases, the result is discrimination against the poor. Nurses and social workers should be trained to counsel abortion patients, and good birth control information should be included.

Finally, for those who argue that the product of an unwanted pregnancy might be another Darwin or Beethoven, I would answer that it is more likely that it will be an Oswald or an Eichmann. Countless geniuses have already been snuffed out because of ignorance, indifference, poverty, malnutrition, preventable disease, etc. Even if unwanted pregnancy could be correlated with better-than-average offspring, would we *force* women to breed this way?

In sum, if the men in charge of the world can't make child rearing attractive enough to women, then the race doesn't deserve to go on. Forcing women to bear children is uncivilized. The nation and the world do not need to mass-produce babies any more—quite the contrary. It has been said that if men bore the children, or if women controlled the legislatures, there would be no laws against abortion. I think there would be laws against compulsory pregnancy.

REFERENCES

1. B. Pasamanick. Epidemiologic Investigations of Some Prenatal Factors in the Production of Neuropsychiatric Disorders. In P. H. Hoch and J. Zubin (eds.), *Comparative Epidemiology of the Mental Disorders.* New York: Grune and Stratton (1961).
2. Innes H. Pearse and Lucy H. Crocker. *The Peckham Experiment.* London: George Allen and Unwin, Ltd. (1943), p. 11.
3. E. J. Lieberman. Reserving a Womb: A Case for the Small Family. *American Journal of Public Health 60:*87-92, January 1970.
4. Group for the Advancement of Psychiatry. *The Right to Abortion: A Psychiatric View.* New York. (1969).

Chapter **9**

Health Insurance
for Abortion Costs:
A Survey

Charlotte F. Muller

Most states still permit abortion only when the life of the pregnant woman is threatened. In only three states is abortion a procedure which may be legally and freely decided upon by a woman and her physician. Nevertheless, the momentum with which restrictive abortion laws are being reformed or repealed* indicates that legal access will soon cease to play the central role in keeping the medically poor from obtaining safe abortion services, services that the more economically privileged could often buy via the route of psychiatric certification. The illegal

Adapted from Health Insurance for Abortion Costs: A Survey, *Family Planning Perspectives, 2,* No. 4, and *Inquiry, 7,* No. 3. Reprinted with permission of *Family Planning Perspectives* and *Inquiry.*

*Since 1967 (and as of September 1, 1970) 12 states had reformed their abortion laws (Arkansas, California, Colorado, Delaware, Georgia, Kansas, Maryland, New Mexico, North Carolina, Oregon, South Carolina and Virginia. Three other states permit abortion on grounds broader than threat to the life of the pregnant woman (Alabama and Massachusetts: "health"; Mississippi: "forcible rape"). Three states repealed their restrictive abortion laws in 1970 (New York, Alaska and Hawaii); one other state legislature (Maryland) repealed its liberal reform law but was overridden by a governor's veto. A number of courts, federal and state, have declared abortion laws unconsitutional (including courts in Wisconsin, Pennsylvania, Texas, South Dakota, Illinois, Michigan, California and Georgia—the latter two rulings affecting liberal reform laws), and cases are pending in a number of other states (including Minnesota, New Jersey, Missouri and Oregon), and are contemplated elsewhere. Courts in only two states (Louisiana and Massachusetts) thus far have upheld the constitutionality of restrictive abortion laws. A Federal District Court ruling holding the old District of Columbia law unconstitutional has been appealed and is docketed in the U.S. Supreme Court, which has asked the parties to brief a number of jurisdictional questions having to do with whether they should decide the case.

market, although not well-studied, appears to have its class lines too: the price of a qualified (although legally nonconforming) practitioner's care averages about $1,000(1)—a price clearly prohibitive to many. The methods of interrupting a pregnancy to which the poor have recourse, consequently, have been crude, painful, and often perilous.

With legal access likely to be attained soon in most states, the issue of financial access becomes more salient. Maximum availability of legal abortion services is desirable to society not only to bring about equal distribution of human welfare among those who have a given need but also to assure each child who is born an opportunity for wholesome growth with welcoming parents(2).

For those who receive welfare assistance, costs for legal abortion should be reimbursable under Title XIX of the Social Security Act (Medicaid). This, indeed, appears to be the case in such cities as San Francisco, San Diego, Baltimore, and New York where hospitals to which the poor have access are willing to perform the procedure and where there is some advocate structure to which a woman can turn to establish her eligibility promptly before the pregnancy is too far advanced. Such an 'advocate' may be a Planned Parenthood organization, welfare department, social service division of a hospital, or a health department's Maternity and Infant Care project. Such "advocates" are not always available, and there is evidence that where they are not, welfare clients find it difficult or impossible to obtain medical abortions even where restrictive laws have been reformed or repealed. In any case, eligibility under Medicaid has been made progressively more restrictive so that in most states it covers few beyond the welfare group(3). It is thus, even potentially, a source of abortion cost reimbursement for no more than 14 percent of medically indigent(4) women of child-bearing age.

Private health insurance, largely through employer and union groups, covers a much more significant proportion of this population.†
For this reason a survey was undertaken to find out to what degree private insurance is likely to contribute to the financing of legalized

†Eighty percent of persons under 65 are covered by private insurance for hospital costs, 77 percent for surgical costs. (L. S. Reed, "Private Health Insurance, 1968: Enrollment, Coverage, and Financial Experience," *Social Security Bulletin,* December 1969.) Over two-thirds of the company hospital insurance and five-sixths of the surgical insurance for those under 65 was sold through groups. (Source: *1969 Source Book of Health Insurance Data,* Health Insurance Institute, pp. 20, 22.)

abortion, and to identify and assess problems relating to the adaptation of insurance coverage to a procedure which, for the first time, is likely soon to become widely and legally accessible.

Specifically, it was anticipated that consumer groups (including union memberships) might re-examine their bargaining priorities, that individuals choosing a policy, including group members, could consider in so doing what goes into adequate abortion coverage, and that sellers of coverage might be alerted to possibilities of marketing an improved benefit for which, experience indicates, a lively demand is likely to be expressed. Finally, the identification of financial needs not likely to be met by insurance is the first step towards specific efforts to include abortion in public systems for delivery of health care.

It is difficult to develop completely accurate information on contract benefits under private insurance. Over 700 companies are writing health insurance today. Not only may each of these have its own "standard" contract, but each writes a great many variations for the diverse groups making up its market. Not only do dollar amounts differ, but so do a host of provisions relating to eligibility, waiting periods, duration of benefits and other contract features.

As a practical way of getting ready and reliable, even if incomplete, information, letters were addressed to presidents of the 13 companies which are known as leaders in the writing of group health benefits. (Two leading West Coast companies were included, without concern for their specific rank, to assure regional variation.) The letter requested the maternity portion of the contract for the five largest group policies written by the company, and referred specifically to provisions concerning abortion and to features affecting this coverage, such as waiting periods. Other contract portions which might be referred to in the description of maternity benefits, such as hospital benefits and surgical fee schedules, were also requested.

All the companies replied, although one withheld all requested information on grounds of "policy" and merely discussed future plans and implications of present legal changes. The remaining 12 companies sent the actual contracts, excerpts, or summaries, or a standard contract with an explanation.* One company digested coverage of its 11 largest

*These companies were Equitable Life, Massachusetts Mutual Life, New York Life, John Hancock Mutual Life, Aetna Life & Casualty, Travelers, Metropolitan, Pacific Mutual, Connecticut General, Prudential, Occidental Life of California and CNA Insurance.

groups for the study and all this information was included. The volume of health insurance business represented by the 12 responding firms was over $4 billion in 1968(5).

In some cases a company's five largest groups represented millions of workers and family members, and in other cases, thousands, since even large insurance companies vary their contracts for divisions and occupations within a firm. In all, 10,751,300 persons were represented by the replies received from the 12 responding insurance companies.

Information was also collected with the aid of the National Association of Blue Shield Plans for Blue Shield contracts representing 45,465,104 persons and for Blue Cross contracts in areas totalling 23,557,334 persons (these figures are not additive).

Both group and individual practice service plans and indemnity insurance are represented in information, included here, on the federal employees' health benefit plan for almost eight million persons. Also presented is coverage under CHAMPUS, the program for armed service personnel and their dependents. Finally, three self-insured union plans in New York City with covered populations estimated at 211,500 were studied. The numbers are cited to suggest the size of the insured population about which there is some information, even though it was not feasible to capture the variations in the group contracts affecting millions more, let alone all of the variations in the groups included in this survey.*

Since information was requested from large companies about large groups (group size implying superior bargaining power of the consumers), the benefit provisions may well be more favorable to consumers than would be typical for group insurance as a whole.

Abortion coverage, where it exists, is generally found within the maternity provisions of group health contracts. About three-fifths of persons covered by basic hospital-surgical, supplementary, and comprehensive major medical plans of commercial carriers in 1966 were in plans with a maternity benefit for employees and dependents. The most common form uses a single maximum applicable to either hospital or surgical expense. In comprehensive major medical policies, maternity

---

*Similar limitations apply to Blue Cross data since only 23 basic certificates (out of 75 plans) specifically mention abortion, whether in order to include it, exclude it, or set restrictions on the benefit. Also, 17 of 72 Blue Shield plans not replying to a national survey by the National Association of Blue Shield Plans are excluded from the data in this report.

benefit provisions do not usually require an initial payment by the patient or any patient share in the cost (coinsurance). The usual maximum is under $300(6).

Benefits in 1967 (based on a one day claims survey) met 69.3 percent of maternity expense for claimants (71.5 percent for hospital care and 66.5 percent for surgery)(7).

FINDINGS: COMMERCIAL COVERAGE FOR ABORTION

Among the 12 responding commercial companies, one company flatly excluded abortion in four of its five leading group plans and for the one group where abortion was allowed only hospital expenses were covered. The remaining 11 companies answered "yes" to the question "Is abortion covered in commercial group contracts?" In general, however, they added a "but." The "but" meant one or more of the following:

Coverage may not be specified in the contract itself.

Single women may not be covered.

Daughters of the insured may not be covered.

A waiting period may be applied to those women who are covered by the contract.

The benefits may be restricted to a hospital.

The size of the benefits may be less than current fees or hospital charges. Ancillary charges in hospital may be subject to a maximum.

Major medical insurance may not apply to pregnancy.

Different ways of computing the benefit make it difficult to compare insurance policies as to adequacy.

"YES—BUT" SPELLED OUT

Specific mention of abortion in the contract offers more assurance of coverage than language which requires administrative extension in order to apply. Examples of the latter are "miscarriage," "surgery as a result of pregnancy," "expense . . . in connection with pregnancy," and "obstetrical services rendered by the Physician."

Maternity coverage under which abortion is subsumed was generally available to female employees regardless of marital status, but in two companies the pattern was to cover only those employees who had a husband insured as a dependent, and in some plans maternity benefits were restricted to wives of covered employees. Three companies of the 12 responding included *any* dependent, such as a child, in the maternity coverage of some groups. One of these three, however, warned that this was not "usual" in its group business. One company covered unmarried dependents in the three of the five group contracts cited, the contracts with dependents included numbering close to one million persons. Many of this company's other large customer groups have this coverage.

The more common practice in group health policies was to exclude child dependents, which was a more open situation than the Blue Shield/Blue Cross custom of containing maternity coverage within a family contract that excluded both the newlywed and the unwed from maternity coverage.

All forms of maternity care coverage by the 12 large carriers most commonly stipulated that the pregnancy must have started after insurance became effective. This was the general case for five companies, and for some groups in all other companies.

None of the group policies studied restricted abortion benefits to in-hospital procedures. However, one large company wrote that the claim is not questioned "so long as it is performed by a qualified physician in a licensed hospital." (Until July, 1970, the New York City Blue Shield schedule recognized only in-hospital therapeutic abortions(8) as a covered procedure.) Previously, legal limits on abortion made consideration of out-of-hospital coverage academic; however, this condition is rapidly changing. Whether insurance practice will quickly respond to changes in public health codes as to location is now an open question. Present guidelines of the New York State Department of Health recommend restriction to "a hospital having an obstetrical, gynecological or surgical service" or "a suitably equipped and staffed facility administered by such hospital" or having a hospital affiliation agreement(9). This appears to leave room for satellite abortion centers.

In describing the insurer's liability when an employee leaves covered employment, contract language sometimes appears to tie post-termination eligibility for pregnancy benefits to hospital confinement. This is realistic in relation to delivery but might be unsuitable for abortion.

The inadequacy of abortion benefits is part of the general picture of contract schedule maxima which are exceeded by actual fees. This is true for surgery as a whole but is especially true for conditions connected with pregnancy. It would be ideal if the variation in reported surgical allowances (from $25 on up) for miscarriage or abortion were merely a reflection of variations in regional or class markets for medical care, but the evidence indicates otherwise. Table 1 shows that only five of the 12 responding companies have group contracts reimbursing for abortion at prevailing or usual, customary and reasonable (UCR) fees among some of their offerings. One of these companies explained that the claims department developed its own informal schedule from experience, seeking guidance from knowledgeable physicians as to the "reasonableness" of a claim that exceeded expectations. Commitment to pay "prevailing fees" is interpreted slightly less generously than "reasonable and customary." Full fee reimbursement, however, portends a future financial problem for patients if it invites physicians to raise fees and thus puts upward pressure on premiums, but low schedule amounts place an immediate burden on the patient.

Other benefit inadequacies included: 1) Limits placed on the hospital benefit for *any* procedure in the domain of maternity. (One plan allowed only $100 for hospital expenses, while another allowed up to $200. These are examples of overall maximum sums.) 2) Benefits set at a low daily maximum for room and board charges. Such a limit was not found in most of the plans in this study since full semi-private coverage or a blanket ceiling for hospital and surgical costs for maternity prevailed, but this problem is documented from other sources. Thus, among new group plans tabulated by the health insurance industry in 1969, the average maximum daily hospital room and board benefit (DRB) was between $24 and $27, depending on group size, for employees with basic coverage only, and between $27 and $33 for those with basic *and* major medical coverage. As an example of extreme inadequacy, 16 percent of the basic coverage group had less than $20 benefit(10).

A reporting service listed some recent group plans that cover maternity hospital expense at the same level as other disabilities and that cite a daily maximum which conforms with industry DRB statistics. (For instance, an electrical workers' plan pays $35 a day for room and board; a printers' plan, $27; and a union of operating engineers', $30.)

Although national figures were not available on per diem charges for room and board alone, figures for total costs and revenue per day in

TABLE 1. *Reimbursement for abortion: payment basis, waiting period and eligibility requirements, 12 responding companies*

Company number	Abortion expense reimbursement*	Waiting period for maternity in general	Persons eligible	No. of persons in cited contracts
1	UCR (3);SCHED. (2 groups; in one salaried have BLANKET).	Pregnancy starts while insured.	Employee, wife.	290,000
2	SCHED.	Pregnancy starts while insured.	Employee, dependent.	225,200
3	UCR included in BLANKET (2 groups), SCHED. (two groups).	9 months (4 groups), None (1).	Employee, wife.	166,145
4	All 3 forms in major contracts.	9 months or pregnancy starts while insured.	Employee, wife (1 group). Wife; employee only if she has an insured husband (4).	464,320
5	SCHED.(except for one group: UCR).	Pregnancy starts while insured (2 groups), none (2); 270 days except for miscarriage (1).	Employee, dependent (3 groups), Employee, wife, (2).	328,940
6	SCHED. or BLANKET.	Pregnancy starts while insured (one group has 23 months wait).	Employee, wife.	71,435
7	UCR except group (5) $60.	Pregnancy starts while insured (3 groups), except: return from military service (1).	Employee, dependent (3 groups). Employee, wife (2).	2,090,000

8	$100 for miscarriage; "Regular" if disability or rape.	Pregnancy starts while insured.	Employee, wife.	75,000
9	Not covered.	None (3 groups); 3 months (1), pregnancy starts while insured (1).	Employee, wife.	48,200
10	Majority in BLANKET; minority on SCHED.	Pregnancy starts while insured (Rare: two years, employees only).	Employee, wife.	4,875,000
11	SCHED.	Pregnancy starts while insured.	Employee, wife.	1,200,000
12	SCHED.	Pregnancy starts while insured.	Wife, employee with insured husband.	400,000
Total				10,234,240

*According to: a dollar schedule (SCHED.), prevailing or customary fees (UCR), or as part of maximum sum allowed for any maternity benefits (BLANKET).

hospitals suggest that hospital DRB benefits are inadequate. Expense per patient day in nonfederal short-term hospitals was $61.38 in 1968, and inpatient revenue (for nongovernmental community hospitals) was $56.52. These averages contain a wide interstate variation, with revenue per day varying from a low of $33.69 (Wyoming) to a high of $80 (California)(11). In 1970, hospital benefits went even less far to meet charges, since daily service charges in the Consumers' Price Index rose 11.7 percent in 1969.

A low daily maximum may be combined with an allowance for miscellaneous hospital expense for surgery, and may be expressed as 10, 20, or some other number of times the DRB charge (12). For this reason the DRB maximum is of special interest when maternity is placed on the same basis as other surgical procedures for determining hospital benefits. In the present study, one company used a multiple (20 times) of *actual* room and board charges as the ceiling for miscellaneous hospital services. This offered more protection against variation in costs between hospitals and against cost increases than would either the daily benefit base or an overall maximum for maternity, but was inferior to the full service benefit offered by some carriers.

Although it is the rare abortion case that runs into difficulty and requires an extended stay, together with extra blood, laboratory work, and other services, financial protection against such contingencies should enter into the conception of benefit adequacy. Specific information on major medical protection for pregnancy was not sought (and some policies had no major medical feature); however, returns from five companies (see Table 2) showed one (No. 3) which apparently excluded pregnancy from all groups, and one (No. 7) which excluded pregnancy for some; one (No. 2) which included it for all groups reported on; three (Nos. 1, 5, 7) that did so for one or more groups; one (No. 5) that admitted complications of pregnancy to coverage; and one (No. 7) that did so for severe complications only. Company 2, with the most generous major medical coverage for pregnancy, also included in its basic policy coverage (90 days in hospital) of any sickness to which pregnancy contributed. Unlimited ancillary hospital services for maternity, as offered by Company 3, augmented the coverage along the same lines.

Major medical policies may (like Company 2) favor pregnancy claims by provisions which pay on a per pregnancy basis "without regard to total disability, accumulation period, calendar year, etc." This applies to both supplementary and comprehensive policies.

The difficulty of comparing policies as to adequacy is well illustrated by the coexistence of three methods of payment among the group policies of a single company (No. 6). These are: a blanket sum for maternity; usual charges (UCR) for doctors' services and a flat sum for hospital expense; and a surgical schedule combined with a hospital daily allowance.

BLUE CROSS–BLUE SHIELD COVERAGE

National data indicate that surgical and hospital expense for abortion qualify for coverage in most Blue Cross and Blue Shield plans. However, the number of persons covered is restricted by requirements of family contracts and by waiting periods for maternity benefits. Also, benefits are limited by low dollar ceilings. Furthermore, anomalies exist

TABLE 2. *Definition of dependency and major medical provisions related to pregnancy, five companies* *

Company number	General definition of a dependent†	Does major medical include pregnancy?	Relevant provisions related to major medical coverage
1	Not stated.	Yes (one group).	
2	Spouse, child if under 19, or if disabled. Includes adopted and stepchildren. Students to 21 - 22-23 for extra rate.	Yes.	Sickness to which pregnancy contributed, 90 days in basic.
3	Not stated.	Not stated.	Unlimited ancillary hospital (1,2) for maternity.
5	Spouse, child to age 25 or disabled sponsored dependent if lives with head (one group); to age 19 or 23 if student (one group).	Yes (one group) Complications (2 groups).	
7	Spouse, child to 19-23 (2 groups), 21-25 (2 groups), sponsored dependents (in 2 groups).	Yes—comprehensive policy (2 groups); Yes (1 group); Severe complications (in 2 groups): No (in 1 group).	365 days for complications of pregnancy.

*Other companies: items omitted or no major medical.

†Company 6 includes children to age 23.

where Blue Cross and Blue Shield provisions are not coordinated. For example, Chicago and Dallas Blue Shield cover abortion, but the Blue Cross plans in those areas do not.

An important change occurred in June, 1970, when the New York City Blue Cross plan announced extension of abortion coverage to single women and unmarried dependent children in families covered by community-rated* contracts, or about half of the metropolitan area membership of some eight million. A similar benefit was made available to those who were in experience-rated** groups through purchase of a rider at extra cost(13). The Blue Shield plan in New York City made a parallel change in its coverage; however, claims for service rendered in independent facilities meeting criteria of the City Board of Health will be honored, whereas the Blue Cross benefit is confined to hospitals(14). (Physicians' offices do not have access to back-up facilities required by current city standards.)

All Blue Cross plans throughout the U. S. provide maternity benefits with waiting periods of eight to 10 months. Twenty-nine of these plans set no limits on dollars or days in the hospital; 22 others limit stay; and a third group of 22 plans have a dollar maximum, with ceilings of $80 or less in over half of these plans(15).

A survey of the plans listed in the Blue Cross Manual shows that there are 23 that mention abortion. These have a membership of 24,917,000, as of March 31, 1970(16). Among these 23 plans, three that exclude abortion represent 6.2 million members. Among the 20 plans that include abortion, eight waive a waiting period if delivery would have occurred after the usual maternity waiting period; three specify a waiting period and one exempts abortion from a waiting period if both husband and wife are subscribers. In four plans the usual ceiling for maternity expense does not apply to abortion. There are also four plans in which a maximum number of benefit days is stated(17).

Obstetrical benefits are universal in Blue Shield plans throughout the United States but are limited to employee and wife under a husband-wife or family contract. Twenty-one plans (of 72) cover prenatal care and 25 plans cover postnatal care. Service benefits

*Community rating is a single premium schedule applicable to members of the population.

**Experience rating adjusts a group's premium cost on the basis of past losses on claims for a specific covered group and implies lower cost where utilization has been low.

(payment of all costs) for maternity are rare(18). Allowances are low relative to charges, ranging from $50 to $157.50 per day, the mode being $70-79(19). The waiting period is usually nine months, the range being seven to 11 months.

When surveyed about coverage for abortion by the National Association of Blue Shield Plans in April, 1970, 55 Blue Shield Plans replied. Of these, 51 include abortion coverage. (The four 'excluding' plans represent a quarter of a million persons and the 51 'including' plans, 45,465,000)(20). Of the 51 plans, 24 pay on the basis of a dollar schedule benefit; six pay "usual, customary and reasonable charges;" seven pay according to a combination of these two methods; and for 14 plans the basis of payment could not be ascertained.

FEDERAL EMPLOYEES' PLANS

The federal employees' health benefits program, which included 7,816,965 persons in the calendar year 1967(21), covers maternity without waiting periods in all plans offered. Also covered are "any expenses in connection with legal abortions that are medically necessary(22).

However, family coverage is required in many of the plans. The exceptions are two of the group practice plans, Kaiser and Health Insurance Plan of Greater New York (HIP). Family coverage usually implies limitation to employees and wives. For plans that use a dollar schedule for surgical procedures, applicable allowances range from $40 to $134, depending on plan, place, and whether high or low option. Substantial partial payment toward hospitalization is required of the patient in the Kaiser and Group Health Association plans. HIP provides the most complete financial protection.

Another federal health program, the Civilian Health and Medical Program of the Uniformed Services (CHAMPUS) also covers abortion, so long as state law permits. It would appear, however, that abortions may be performed "in military facilities of the United States without regard to local state laws"(23).

Wives and unmarried daughters to age 21 (23 if students) are included without a waiting period. The dependent of an active duty member pays the first $25 or $1.75 per day of hospitalization, whichever is greater; the dependent of a retired member or the surviving dependent of a deceased member pays 25 percent of charges. In each

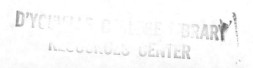

case CHAMPUS pays the remaining costs if based on customary charges to the public (hospital) and reasonable fees (doctors). Of the covered population of six million, 1.5 million are wives and 2.3 million are children, but the age distribution of the children is not known(24).

EXAMPLES OF COVERAGE IN SELF-INSURED PLANS

Three self-insured union plans were studied; Local 1 of the Dining Room Employees Union, Local 1199 Drug and Hospital Employees Union, and the 65 Security Plan of the Retail, Wholesale and Department Store Union. These were found to share with many of the commercial plans limitation to employees or wives, a mixture of service (UCR) and schedule coverage for both hospital and surgical components of care, and the requirement that pregnancy start while insured. The Local 1199 plan is of special interest because the trustees, responding to New York State's repeal of its abortion law, approved the following benefits for abortion, effective September, 1970: hospitalization $100, "miscarriage" $75, accompanied by one week's disability benefits under the effective plan.

In Local 1 of the Dining Room Employees Union, employees and wives are eligible for maternity benefits provided pregnancy starts "while eligible for full benefits." For miscarriage or abortion, regular hospital benefits at full charges for semi-private rates for 21 days are payable, starting with the date of termination of pregnancy. It would appear that $8 a day for 10 days would be paid for care before this date. A schedule maximum of $50 is payable for miscarriage, which can be interpreted to mean abortion.

The 65 Security Plan has maternity benefits for employees who were in a covered shop 10 months before taking maternity leave. Wives of members are under the same provisions as female employees, if the member was covered for 10 months before delivery. Medical care is on a service (UCR) basis. For miscarriage or abortion hospital benefits are provided on the same basis as general illness.

In the Local 1199 self-insured plan, the insured (wife, or employee regardless of marital status) is eligible if conception occurs after the employer has made contributions for comprehensive benefits for 30 days. Hospital expense, while limited to $150 for a delivery, is unlimited for other procedures, both as to days and as to any maximum daily charge. The doctor's allowance for "miscarriage" with dilation and curettage is $75. Pregnancy conditions are eligible for major medical benefits only if there are complications.

DISCUSSION

The kind of benefits a consuming group gets depends ultimately on what it is prepared to pay for. Competition, including choice of independent service plans and of self-insured plans, helps keep options open. Consumers have no need to feel constrained by old philosophies or categories so long as buying power backs up their selections. The case of abortion can be viewed in this light. There is no reason why coverage could not extend to all single female employees (including the divorced and separated as well as those never previously married), and to the unmarried dependent children of an insured father or mother.

"Dependent," as used in group health insurance, includes adopted, step, and foster children, and, in general, unmarried and economically dependent children sharing a household with the insured head. The age limit is 18 or 19 years, but this is frequently extended to 21 or 22 years and more for students (one company is now changing over to age 26) and there is no age limit for a disabled child. Extension of abortion coverage to all these dependents would take in a large portion of the younger group at risk. Although in the past the young patient has not always shared her needs with her family, legalization may partially change this. It is interesting to contemplate how the security of knowing that the family's insurance entitlements can be applied to the young women members in time not only of need but of distress would add to family strength.

There is no reason why coverage could not be written without a waiting period. The view sometimes stated to justify maternity waiting periods, namely, that the insurance mechanism is misused when it finances a planned event, would surely not apply to the unwanted pregnancy. Moreover the liability is less than for delivery. General surgical schedules now include gynecological procedures, such as dilation and curettage, that are not related to pregnancy (for which dependent daughters are commonly eligible). A reduction in claims for dilation and curettage can be expected as a result of legalizing abortion. Abortion services can be assimilated to surgery and made a full benefit (at "reasonable and customary charges") as surgery now is in the superior group plans. Or it can be reimbursed at full charges, as a desirable "special benefit," even if surgery in general is left on a dollar schedule. It can be argued that, in general, poverty will be reduced by minimizing all financial barriers to the prevention of unwanted births.

Protection is best assured when abortion is mentioned specifically in the contract and when the statement of the abortion benefit is separated from references to the diagnosis and treatment of sickness and injury. (Tying them together leaves open the question of whether pregnancy is a "sickness" and abortion a "treatment" for it.) Since sterilization is covered specifically in 72 Blue Cross and 57 Blue Shield plans, and cosmetic surgery in 43 Blue Cross and 19 Blue Shield plans(25), there is ample economic precedent for insurance that is disconnected from such a sickness casualty approach.

Another place for abortion coverage is in the area of preventive services, especially if service is placed on an ambulatory basis. The expansion of ambulatory and preventive coverage has been espoused by the entire insurance industry, and has been realized in some group plans. Inclusion of abortion coverage can give assurance that this service will not only be covered financially but will be provided within the framework of a program of preventive medicine.

The social and humanitarian implications of good insurance benefits for abortion are almost too obvious to mention. Whereas these considerations lead into a case for public sector intervention (as, a system of free abortion centers), the insurance market is also a societal device to bring about desired results—both in the sense that the market is dependent on collective bargaining established under public law, and on tax privileges for the employer contribution which is entailed, and in the sense that the public's preferences and even its knowledgeable buying and in the consequent adaptation of types of services or products offered to effective demand reflecting informed choice.

As in proposals for extending health insurance generally, a case can be made for public subsidy of abortion coverage for those at higher risk who are less able to pay. Regardless of one's choice of philosophies, it would appear that adequate abortion insurance would have a strong market, if carriers are willing to pick up the challenge.

THE FUTURE

What do insurance companies actually say about the future? Of the 12 who responded to our query, one is evaluating the insurance aspects of abortion reform legislation. Another is considering its future claims policy with regard to "elective" abortion but is now paying all claims in states that have legalized abortion. A third company says it is reviewing its liability for cases which are "not medically necessary." A threat to the life or health of the pregnant woman, or pregnancy resulting from incest or forcible or statutory rape is grounds of "necessity," whereas a case "where the child is unwanted" is not. Still another company would distinguish between such cases, not as to *whether* it would pay, but *how much:* "regular" benefits are applicable to an abortion classed as "necessary," i.e., full charges as distinct from a maternity indemnity. Predicting a marked increase in utilization, this last company is considering offering only a limited benefit "until we can develop some meaningful statistics on this new exposure." Still another carrier states: "We have every intention of continuing to cover, even though the exposure will be somewhat greater."

THE COSTS OF COVERING ABORTIONS

A figure which can be used as the basis for the computation of premium cost—an estimated 28.9 abortions per 1,000 women in the child-bearing ages—is derived from calculations involving the rates for live births, fetal deaths, and abortions.

Besides utilization rates, the other necessary element in determining financing requirements is price. The price of abortions in the past has varied over a wide range, a range that is now likely to narrow with a more competitive market, even though it appears that access problems in states with reform laws are far from solved(26). A narrower range will facilitate design of an adequate benefit, and the accompanying actuarial predictions.

However, a surgical benefit within the range of current schedules can be made available at once *without prohibitive cost.* A benefit of $100 would require a pure premium of $2,890 in a group of 1,000 women age 15-44, or $2.89 per capita—less if the cost is shared among the males. From such beginnings, further experimentation should be feasible. A $200 benefit yields a pure premium cost of $5.98.

New insurance benefits, whether public or private, add effective demand to the market and encourage physicians to raise fees. Such fee increases may thwart efforts to assure payment of full medical costs of abortion through insurance. Recognition of the social benefits to be gained from a reduction of unwanted pregnancy may sustain a movement for alternative sources of supply (such as a health department center or special clinics) as a way out of fee practice in a hospital setting. It may be desirable to recognize such possibilities explicitly in group insurance contracts both to assure honoring of the surgical claim and to cover any institutional charges, as, for use of a recovery room in a clinic facility. One way of doing this is to refer to any facilities licensed by a state health department for abortion services, without narrowly specifying the type of facility. If the anticipated increase in the number of abortions demanded materializes, the flexibility gained by non-hospital financial coverage will be useful.

A MODEL INSURANCE PROVISION

What then, should consumer groups, individuals, union staffs, and public officials dealing with health benefits on behalf of an insured population look for in purchasing abortion expense coverage? First of all, the benefit should be specified in the body of the contract or in a rider; it should not be dependent on administrative interpretation of contract wording such as "miscarriage," "pregnancy," "obstetrics," or "maternity." Benefits should be noncancelable. Adequate coverage of eligible females should include employed women and wives of workers without requiring that they hold a family or maternity contract. Unmarried dependent girls up to the maximum feasible age the group can afford should also be included. (The age of 25 or 26 for students is realistic in terms of present educational requirements in many professional careers elected by young women.) The top age of dependents for an abortion benefit can be higher than the maximum age of dependents for general medical or hospital benefits.

Coverage without a waiting period is the ideal. Short of this, the less extended the waiting period the better the group coverage against risk of expense. Subjection of any subgroup, such as unmarried dependents or single working women, to a specially long waiting period is an impairment of coverage.

The important thing about location of service is that an insurance contract should not be more restrictive than community health standards prescribe. In view of the rapid changes being made with respect to legally permitted location of service, the contract should include both in-hospital and out-of-hospital benefits. It may be necessary to check general clauses defining acceptable institutions, practitioners, and what is a covered illness or condition, to be sure locational restrictions, if any, do not carry over to abortion.

Extension of major medical benefits to abortion services protects against catastrophic rather than ordinary expense; it is a desirable feature to include and should not be financially unwieldy.

The question of the size of benefits is perhaps the most difficult one to resolve. A financially adequate benefit is likely to be expensive, but a limited benefit, although useful in establishing a commitment to cover, contributes to restriction of access. Spreading the cost over an entire group, rather than leaving large out-of-pocket expense to the patient is appropriate to abortion service. Full payment of basic and ancillary hospital charges and of physician fees is the only type of coverage which would qualify as ideal. A "usual and customary fee" approach might be protected by a device that would activate "self-discipline" by physicians (such as a medical society review committee) or initiate outside discipline and publicizing of excesses by group purchases in the community.

If a contract requires the patient to pay a certain amount, it is less burdensome to her if such payment is defined in terms of dollars instead of a percentage. A standard way of expressing benefits, such as full payment of all charges (basic and ancillary hospital expense and medical fees), subject to a patient contribution of X dollars and within an *overall* maximum of Y dollars, would facilitate comparison of prices and values of competing plans. An overall maximum provides more flexibility than separate maxima for the hospital and medical components.

A punitive approach to personal behavior is irrelevant in coping with poverty and inadequate child rearing. The birth of the unwanted child is prevented by abortion. Sooner or later, we will have to settle on a strong insurance approach to a service that is small in its ordinary details, rarely of catastrophic consequences medically, and laden with long-run social impact in terms of population and poverty.

REFERENCES

1. A. F. Guttmacher. *Birth Control and Love,* Macmillan, New York, N.Y., 1969, p. 209.
2. C. F. Muller. Socio-Economic Outcomes of Present Abortion Policy, paper delivered at the National Institute of Child Health and Human Development and National Institute of Mental Health, Bethesda, Md., Dec. 15-16, 1969.
3. J. I. Rosoff. *Family Planning, Medicaid and the Private Physician,* Center for Family Planning Program Development, No. 9, New York, N.Y., 1969.
4. G. Varky et al. *Five Million Women,* Planned Parenthood-World Population, New York, N.Y., 1967.
5. Argus Chart of Health Insurance.
6. Based on replies of 56 principal companies in *A Profile of Group Health Insurance in Force in the United States,* Dec. 31, 1966, Health Insurance Association of America, pp. 25, 30.
7. *A Comparison of Group Medical Care Insurance Benefits to Charges,* Health Insurance Association of America, June 1968.
8. *Participating Physicians' Schedule of Allowances and Handbook,* United Medical Service, September 1964, p. 95.
9. State of New York. *Department of Health Hospital Memorandum Series 70-24* , Abortional Acts, May 25, 1970.
10. Health Insurance Institute. *New Group Health Insurance Policies Issued in 1969, Complete Tables,* p. 37.
11. *Hospitals,* Guide Issue, August 1, 1969, pp. 475, 500.
12. *New Group Health Insurance Policies Issued in 1969, Complete Tables,* p. 39.
13. *The New York Times,* June 27, 1970.
14. Communication July 2, 1970 from United Medical Service.
15. L. S. Reed and W. Carr. *Benefit Structure of Private Health Insurance 1968,* Social Security Administration, Office of Research and Statistics, Research Report No. 32, 1970, p. 13.
16. Blue Cross Association. *Blue Cross Enrollment and Utilization Report, First Quarter,* 1970, July 8, 1970.
17. Communication April 14, 1970, from National Association of Blue Shield Plans.
18. Reed and Carr, *op. cit.,* p. 35.

19. *Ibid.,* p. 39.
20. U. S. Social Security Administration. *Research and Statistics Note No. 22-1969, Enrollment and Finances of Blue Cross and Blue Shield Plans, 1968,* December 8, 1969.
21. U. S. Civil Service Commission, Bureau of Retirement and Insurance. *Report for Fiscal Year Ended June 30, 1968,* p. 36.
22. Communication from Solomon Papperman, Chief of Legislative and Policy Division of the U. S. Civil Service Commission, Bureau of Retirement Insurance and Occupational Health, June 11, 1970.
23. *Memorandum for the Surgeons General of the Military Departments,* from Louis M. Rousselot, M. D., Deputy Assistant Secretary for Health and Environment, Department of Defense, July 31, 1970.
24. Communication from Vernon McKenzie, Office of Assistant Secretary of Defense, August 12, 1970.
25. Reed and Carr, *op. cit.,* pp. 14, 41.
26. *The New York Times,* June 8, 1970.

Chapter 10

Abortion:
A Political View

Senator Maurine Neuberger

Stewart Chase once wrote an article called "Purr Words and Slur Words." Examples of the former are: Mother, moonlight, roast beef, balanced budget. Slur words include: Politician, taxes, Communist, turnip, abortion.

Recently a reporter asked me if I had long been associated with the movement to repeal abortion laws, and I told him that I hadn't. When he asked me when I had become interested, I had to stop and think because I have worked in many, many other areas in the field of health. Actually, not until the task force report on family law issued by the Citizens' Advisory Council (April, 1968) on the Status of Women got working on the abortion problem did I really begin to think about it. As Stewart Chase said about purr words and slur words, we all associate to words, and unpleasant images accumulate around a word like "abortion" that conjure up visions of illicit activities, adultery, and scenes in back rooms where those who deal in human misery ply their illegal practices.

In the report, which is quite lengthy, there is one little paragraph of two lines which states: "We are convinced that the right of a woman to determine her own reproductive life is a basic human right. Therefore, the task force recommends repeal of laws making abortion a crime."

While we were working on the report, all sorts of questions came up for discussion: whether women should have the right to manage their own property; whether or not they can lift weights; whether they

Delivered as the keynote address before the California Conference on Abortion, May, 1969.

should work overtime to earn premium pay, etc., but the abortion problem was the one that really attracted attention. My secretary began to phone me in Boston, saying: "We are running out of reports— we are having to have them reprinted. We have a best seller on our hands!"

A few years earlier, I had served on the Status of Women Commission, which was appointed by President Kennedy. Its Chairman was Eleanor Roosevelt, and the Assistant Chairman was Esther Peterson. Mrs. Roosevelt died before we finished our report, and Esther Peterson took over. Our studies of the laws that affect women led us to believe that it was time to talk about abortion laws, but we couldn't get our own Commission to consider such a discussion. It was said that the word "abortion" was verboten; that we couldn't get anything printed about it in government publications. Believing all this, when the task force report came to my desk, I anticipated all sorts of trouble. I expected delays and hours of debate. But not so. What had happened in that interval of a few years? Well, an educational process had been going on, organizations had been at work, and there had been a complete change in the emotional climate. The greatest dissension came, as we studied the task force report, over the proposal to amend the maximum hours law to permit women to work overtime! Very little—there was one minority report—on the abortion report. When somebody said, "Remember before, we couldn't get the government printing office to print it?" I said, "I will contact the Secretary myself." So I called up Secretary of Labor Bill Wirtz and said, "Bill, we are going to have this task force report ready soon." He said, "Fine, go ahead and print it." So here we are, in business.

Legislation conforms to the reality of the times. For instance, speed laws were liberalized to conform to what automobiles were capable of doing and to improved techniques and safer roads; some states even did away with their maximum miles per hour. Divorce laws with phony residence requirements that force people to go to Mexico are being changed. Deans of women would now be burned in effigy if they tried to enforce the campus rules—in your rooms at 8:30 and lights out at ten—that I lived under when I was in college. Yet that kind of discipline didn't make me better educated than the college girls I know today. So times are changing rapidly.

The best analogy that I can think of to the repeal of abortion laws is with the repeal of prohibition. Prohibition did not work despite the fact that it was a constitutional amendment—which meant that support had been given by three-fourths of the States—and in spite of strenuous efforts by officials to enforce it. Actually, there is really more reason for controlling alcohol consumption than for controlling abortion because alcoholism is a disease that causes misery to the victim and psychological injury to his family. Lawyers and legislators say that when there is a substantial difference of opinion as to whether a criminal law is good or not—whether it will work—then one can be sure that it is unworkable and unrealistic. And this is true of laws that prohibit abortions.

How, for instance, does one establish rape? Maybe the sexual act was perfectly agreeable to the girl until she got pregnant. In such cases, the "rape" is rarely reported to the police or even mentioned to the girls' parents unless pregnancy occurs. In many cases, according to lawyers, the use of the word "rape" is highly questionable.

Then, too, abortion is an individual problem, not a government problem. The individual is responsible for the care and upbringing of the child. True, the government will make a token effort, but oh, how little. And there is no substitute, of course, for the atmosphere of a warm home with good family relationships and a wanted child.

Before I left Boston I thought it well to substantiate some of the things that our task force reported because, after all, almost a year had elapsed. I have close associations at the Harvard Medical School, so I called on my friends. One is a leading obstetrician in Boston—I would almost call him a society obstetrician. I said to him, "I want to talk to you about this conference on abortion." He was great. He talked to me at great length, and he told me this story:

Recently, a daughter of a nationally-known insurance executive came in and asked for an abortion. She lives in a Boston suburb where only the so-called best people live. She goes to a good college. She is age 20. And my good friend, Dr. A, said: "What's the matter with you? You are a smart girl. Why don't you take the pill?" And she said, "Well, I did take it for a while, but I read so many articles about its side effects that I was afraid of what might happen." He said: "You didn't stop having intercourse, did you? You mean you didn't know what the side effects of that are?" Oh, he was furious with her. He cited her as one of the rich who *cannot* get an abortion on demand. Many of the rich take their daughters on an "educational" trip to Japan, and that is what the parents of this girl had to do.

I asked another doctor, "Why is the medical profession interested in the legal aspects of so-called criminal abortion?" He replied "Because medicine is shifting from a concern limited to treatment of disease to concern with health, including mental health." When I asked my obstetrician friend how to answer the question about psychosis, neurosis, and psychological damage, he replied, "I have never had a married or unmarried patient on whom I performed an abortion who wasn't damned relieved." He went on to say that abortion doesn't make a woman neurotic, but an unwanted pregnancy may.

What, I asked, would doctors like to see in an abortion law if we must have a law? He answered: One, that abortions shouldn't be done by bunglers, which—as he said—is good trade union practice as well as sound medicine. Two, to use the Model Penal Code of the American Law Institute as a basis for a new nation-wide abortion law. To it should be added a clause that would permit taking into consideration the life conditions of the mother, such as having too many children already, low income, or poor family relationships. Because, of course, a woman may be perfectly capable of bearing a fifth or sixth or seventh child, but what will bearing them do to her and to the children she already has if she hasn't the money, space, time, or energy to take proper care of them, or—even worse—doesn't want them. What is worse than an unwanted child?

Then there is the plight of the unmarried woman, especially the one who can't finance a trip to Japan, or doesn't dare tell her family. Perhaps she could marry the father of her child, but that might end in an unhappy marriage and an early divorce. Or she could go through the anguish of bearing the child and putting him up for adoption, a course of action that is far more likely to cause guilt feelings and psychological problems than an abortion early in pregnancy. Finally, she can have an abortion—if she can find a physician who will recommend an abortionist.

Any women, whether married or not, should be able to secure a safe abortion at a reasonable fee by a licensed and competent physician. Perhaps because I live right in the heart of a college community face-to-face with the facts, my outlook on this subject tends to be broad and forgiving. I was head of a house at Radcliffe and talked to a lot of girls and I understand their problems.

I believe that there is a plausible moral argument for allowing abortions. The criterion should not be a theory of whether the fetus is a human being during those early weeks of pregnancy, but the mother's desire for the child.

Catholic clergy are aware that the social evils that accompany forced pregnancy far outweigh the potential evil of destroying the fetus. Before I left for this conference I talked with Robert F. Drinan, S.J.* "Father Drinan," I said, "I am going out to California to speak at a conference on abortion, and I am going to quote you." "Fine," he said. "We didn't ask the legislature to pass a law stating that it was illegal and a criminal offense to eat meat on Friday." And, in fact, Father Drinan has suggested repealing the anti-abortion laws.

At this point I must give credit to Alice Rossi of Johns Hopkins University, who presented the professional material that was so persuasive to the task force and to the Council on the Status of Women, and that gave them the fortitude, the courage, and the material and background to recommend repeal of criminal abortion laws. Alice Rossi pointed out to us 1) that the American Law Institute's Model Code leaves untouched the vast majority of women who now secure illegal abortions, and 2) that the Model Code means more committees to review abortion cases, involving among other things the loss of precious time while the committee deliberates, and increasing the probability of surgical complications. Mrs. Rossi has pointed out that the Model Code still keeps abortion under the criminal code, although this is true of no other medical procedure. The code satisfies few and discriminates against many, for it sanctions abortions in some cases while saying that abortions in all other cases are immoral.

It reminds me of the cigarette people. I am proud of the fact that I am responsible for the label on cigarette packages which says that it may be hazardous to your health to smoke. But that wasn't part of my bill. My bill called for a label that would say, "Smoking cigarettes may cause death from lung cancer and other diseases." You don't think I could get that through the Congress of the United States, do you? They just weren't willing to face up to it, because the American Tobacco Institute has the most powerful lobby that I have seen in a long time. They fought it to the bitter end. We compromised; we made a start. And for this I will ever be thankful to Robert Kennedy who stood with me on the floor of the Senate and defended even this meager token,

*Father Drinan, formerly dean of the Boston College Law School, is now a member of Congress from Mass. For a recent statement of his views, see Strategy on Abortion, *America* (4 February 1967): 177-179. Ed.

because this was the first time the great government of the United States had ever taken a stand in this area. Others wanted such a strong-termed label that they wouldn't even vote for this bill. But when the bill that we passed expired and was up for repassage, who was there supporting the label on the cigarette package? Why, the American Tobacco Institute, because they were so afraid that we would pass a bill that would make a more frightening label mandatory.

We have only to look at the statistics in Catholic countries to know that there is a vast discrepancy between practice and doctrine. We have heard about the charter flights to London from the Continent. Where do you think these women come from? They come from France and Italy to get their abortions in London.

The laws are supposed to act as a deterrent to extramarital sex relations, but in fact they don't. Our anti-abortion laws are simply forcing people to be lawbreakers. Recently, the Supreme Court addressed itself to problems of personal freedom, holding that the Government may not interfere with personal rights which are, in many ways, less fundamental than this one.

I want to tell you this: Repeal will not come from the legislators, where the political pressures are so great, but from the courts. All legislators are subject to great fears which condition the basic processes of democracy. Thus very often politicians do not do what they want to do, but what they must (or think they must) do in order to keep their power. A member of Congress does not vote or speak without weighing the possible repercussions and recriminations of his words. If he misjudges the reaction of his constituents, he will not again be elected by them.

Because this great fear hangs over every politician, we understand and realize how in every one of us there comes a moment of rationalization. When I first went into the legislative body, I said, "I don't owe anybody anything. I have nothing to fear. I am going to speak out. I am going to say what I think on every subject." And I did. But there were times, because I knew I was going to run for reelection, that this was very difficult, and there were times when I could see what my colleagues were going through. I remember working very closely with Senator Lister Hill of Alabama for increased funds for research in cancer and other diseases. The work was successful and the budget of the National Institutes of Health went up and up. But when Senator Hill came up for reelection, he voted against the Civil Rights Law. One night I said to my husband, "What's wrong with Lister? He's been in Congress 35 years. He's an elder statesman. Why doesn't he just say, 'I am sick and tired of my State of Alabama being at the bottom of everything, and I am going to quit this foolishness'?" And my husband replied, "But he would be defeated in Alabama, and we need him."

So the legislator votes according to his own preference when there is no particular reason why he shouldn't. That is, when any powerful force that he is amenable to, such as the President, or a newspaper, or the Sierra Club, or the American Medical Association, has expressed an opinion that coincides with his own.

But think of him at bay: one group urging him to vote for the oil depletion allowance; the other side promising retaliation at the polls if he does. He cannot vote either way without alienating support. In such a case he usually votes to maintain the status quo. He knows the oil companies will note how he voted, and he also knows that the public forgets. Finally, he may even vote against his own conviction when he finds that to do otherwise would cost him support. For instance, some legislators voted to have no birth control information disseminated by the Agency for International Development (AID). Some, having read the report on cigarette smoking and aware that it can cause emphysema and early death, still voted for the tobacco lobby. Legislators do not lead their constituents in bringing about social change. They follow. Current abortion laws are archaic, unworkable, and discriminatory, but they will remain so until pressure is brought to bear.

In conclusion, I reflect on my long activity in behalf of the status of women. Men make the laws. Do they still believe that women are their chattels? Do they subconsciously feel that women are not virtuous? Men make these laws because they believe in retribution: "Abortion is a crime and you must suffer the punishment for becoming pregnant if you are poor or unmarried or already have a large family."

Who decides when life begins? Men, who have never borne nor suckled a child. Who drew up the laws declaring that a woman has no control over the use of her own body? The inseminators. Who sees that these laws are sustained? Men. For what reasons? In their terms: for the sake of the soul, for the preservation of the family, for the good of society, the economy, the state, the wars of conquest. But whose society? Whose markets? Whose state? Whose wars? Certainly not women's.

Through thousands of years the laws that govern the lives of women have been written by men. That man should be the master of his body was never questioned. For many years men have been able to walk into a drug store in any town and buy contraceptives; but a woman—God forbid. She is a vessel to be filled, a field to be planted: such is the natural law, such is the will of God!

What we want is the right for a woman to have an abortion on request; the right to have a life in which she can bear *wanted* children. In the last analysis it is the right of a woman to decide, and is a private matter between herself and her doctor. Let's not have any more committees.

Chapter 11

Unwanted Children

Carl Reiterman

The first question which needs to be asked in relation to unwanted children is, unwanted by whom? The possible answers to this question resemble the set of answers to a multiple-choice question. In the order of their proximity to the mother of the child, they are:

1. The mother.
2. The father.
3. Both of the above.
4. Society.
5. All of the above.

It is important to specify that a responsible answer to our question requires the consideration of at least five alternatives. But even a cursory reading of existing literature on the subject of unwanted children reveals a marked tendency to view the status of the child as determined primarily—if not exclusively—by the mother, sometimes by the father, but seldom by the broader interests of society. If, however, the problems generated by unwanted children are essentially societal, then the interests of society must be seen as having at least equal importance to the judgments of the mother and/or the father.

What, for example, is the significance of the 58,000 babies born to "child" mothers 12-19 years of age in California in 1964?(1) Undoubtedly some were "wanted" by their mothers—especially at the upper end of the age range—and even by their fathers. But, clearly, a large proportion—especially at the lower end of the age range—were wanted neither by their mothers, their fathers, nor by society. Again, studies of California marriages reveal a substantial percentage of premarital pregnancy in marriages between two high school students. For teenage brides in general, the incidence of premarital pregnancy varies between 30 and 50 percent. A major cause of school dropouts in California is premarital pregnancy, sometimes followed by hasty marriage(2). Some of the social costs involved are indicated by the nearly 500,000 children supported, as of May 1966, by California's Aid to Families with Dependent Children program. Eighty percent of these children were under 13 years of age. Sixty-nine percent of the 159,000 families involved in this program were families with estranged parents, and of these families, 46 percent involved children whose parents had never married. Finally, of intact families receiving public assistance in California, 60 percent have six or more members(3).

At the national level, Freedman, Whelpton, and Campbell— reporting in 1959 their findings from interviews with 2,713 white married women between the ages of 18 and 39 who were selected to represent some 17 million wives in the American population as of March 1955—found that 16 percent of the most recent pregnancies were not wanted by the wife, the husband, or both:

> The probability that the most recent pregnancy was unwanted by husband, wife, or both increases rapidly with the number of pregnancies—from 6 percent for first pregnancies to 62 percent among ninth or later pregnancies. Even among couples who had only four pregnancies, 1 in 4 did not want the last. Once a couple has the two, three, or four children commonly considered the ideal number, the likelihood that either the husband or the wife will not want another pregnancy increases rapidly. Partly because of the direct relation between the number of pregnancies and duration of marriage, the proportion of couples with unwanted last pregnancies rises from 3 percent for couples married less than 5 years to 22 percent for those married 15 years or longer(4).

Although the Freedman, Whelpton, and Campbell study did not survey the attitudes of nonwhites, the U. S. Department of Health, Education, and Welfare has reported that a 1960 study revealed that, for the United States as a whole, 17 percent of white families, and 31 percent of nonwhite families, had excess fertility.* Not surprisingly,

*"Excess fertility" is a term used by demographers when either husband or wife or both did not want another child at the time of the last conception.

families with low levels of educational attainment and low income had the highest rates of excess fertility(5).

ILLEGITIMACY

Bronislaw Malinowski has specified that "among the conditions which define conception as a sociologically legitimate fact there is one of fundamental importance. The most important moral and legal rule concerning the physiological side of kinship is that no child should be brought into the world without a man—and one man at that—assuming the role of sociological father, that is, guardian and protector, the male link between the child and the rest of the community"(6). And Kingsley Davis has noted that "the public disapproval of illegitimacy constitutes an integral and necessary part of the social system"(7). Yet, during the 25-year period between 1940 and 1965, the estimated number of illegitimate births in the United States more than tripled, from 89,500 in 1940 to 291,200 in 1965(8). California's contribution to these totals cannot be determined accurately, since California neither reports illegitimate births to the federal government nor records legitimacy on the birth certificate(9). A recent study, however, concluded that of a representative sample of 18,125 California live biths in 1966, 9.3 percent, or almost one in ten, were probably illegitimate(10). This may be compared with the latest available estimate for the United States as a whole, based on a 50-percent sample of births, of 7.7 percent of all births in 1965(11).

Illegitimate births, of course, should be distinguished from illegitimate pregnancies. Not all premarital conceptions result in illegitimate births. In a substantial proportion of cases the couple marries before the birth of the child, and the child is registered as legitimate. A survey conducted by the Bureau of the Census in 1959 indicated that the proportion of legitimate births conceived premaritally has increased substantially over the last fifty years and, especially for white women, during the last twenty-five years prior to the survey. For example, 8 percent of white women first married during 1940-1944 had a first birth within 8 months of marriage. For white women first married during 1955-1959, the proportion had doubled, to 16 percent. The proportion of nonwhite women giving birth to the first child within 8 months of marriage increased in every marriage cohort covered by the study, beginning with 11.8 percent in 1900-1909 and increasing to 41.3 percent in 1950-1959(12).

Although teenagers have the lowest illegitimacy rates (number of illegitimate births per 1,000 unmarried women 15-44 years of age) among women under 35 years of age, more than 40 percent of all illegitimate children are born to mothers 15-19 years of age (123,200 in 1965). A recent report submitted to the Bay Area Social Planning Council concluded that more than 5,600 illegitimate births occur annually in the San Francisco Bay Area, some 10.8 percent of all births in the area, with about half of the illegitimate births occurring to mothers under 20 years of age(13). Because of the proportion of all illegitimate births attributed to teenage mothers, the age structure of the population becomes an important factor, as stressed by Clark Vincent's observation that "the number of thirteen-to-seventeen-year-old unwed mothers in 1970 can be almost double the 1950 number, without any increase in the proportion of all thirteen-through-seventeen-year-old females becoming pregnant out of wedlock." The explanation, as Vincent points out, is purely demographic:

> During the depression years between 1933 and 1937, only approximately 5.25 million females were born. But almost ten million females were born between 1953 and 1957, and they will be the thirteen-through-seventeen-year-olds in 1970(14).

Teenage mothers, however, produce less than half of all illegitimate births. Continuing along the line of Vincent's logic, and assuming that age-specific illegitimacy rates were to continue at their 1965 levels and that the proportion of unmarried women in each age group remains constant, the number of illegitimate births that will occur in the relatively near future can be projected on the basis of the *number* of women at risk. Projections based on the stated assumptions indicate that the number of unmarried women of reproductive age will increase from approximately 12,459,000 in 1965 to approximately 16,173,000 in 1980. The number of illegitimate births would increase correspondingly from the estimated 291,200 in 1965 to 403,000 by 1980(15).

REFERENCES

1. State of California. *Population Study Commission: Report to the Governor.* Berkeley, California: State of California Department of Public Health (1967), p. 45.
2. *Ibid.*
3. *Ibid,* pp. 26, 45-46.
4. Ronald Freedman, Pascal K. Whelpton, and Arthur A. Campbell. *Family Planning, Sterility, and Population Growth.* New York: McGraw-Hill (1959), pp. 10, 75.
5. U. S. Department of Health, Education, and Welfare. *Social Development* (no date available), p. 33.
6. Parenthood, The Basis of Social Structure. Pp. 113-168 in V. F. Calverton and S. D. Schmalhausen (eds.), *The New Generation.* New York: Macauley (1930), p. 137.
7. The Forms of Illegitimacy. *Social Forces 18:*1 (October 1939), p. 89.
8. U. S. Department of Health, Education, and Welfare. *Trends in Illegitimacy: United States, 1940-1965.* Washington, D.C.: U. S. Government Printing Office (February 1968), p. 7. Since the 1940 population of the U. S. was 132 million and the 1965 population almost 195 million, illegitimate births increased at a rate six times the rate of increase for the total population.
9. Although in the 1930's almost every state included a legitimacy item on birth certificates, "during the 1940's . . . a concern for the confidentiality of this item prompted a number of States to remove it." Currently 34 states and the District of Columbia report illegitimacy. Three of the nonreporting states, including the two states with the largest populations—California and New York— together accounted for 21 percent of all births in 1964.(The third state is Massachusetts.) *Trends in Illegitimacy,* p.1. In relation to the nonreporting, nonrecording status of California, Kingsley Davis has remarked: "Is the rising of illegitimacy rate a contributor not only to poverty but to poor child-rearing and swollen welfare rolls? . . . Such questions are not answered, quickly especially since California is gravely deficient in the amount and kinds of information it obtains pertaining to the demographic aspects of its peoples' lives." *Population Study Commission: Report to the Governor,* p. 76.

10.   *Ibid.,* p. 76.
11.   *Trends in Illegitimacy,* p. 8.
12.   *Ibid.,* p. 3.
13.   *San Francisco Chronicle,* 4 January 1968.
14 . *Unmarried Mothers.* New York: Free Press (1961), p. 62. Vincent's
      book is of special interest in the present context, since it was based
      on a study of more than a thousand unmarried mothers in
      Alameda County, California, a county whose birth-control policy
      is reviewed at some length in Carl Reiterman, *Birth-Control Policies
      and Practices in California County Welfare and Health Departments.* Ann
      Arbor, Michigan: University Microfilms (1969).
15.   *Trends in Illegitimacy,* pp. 9-10.

One Hundred and Twenty Children Born After Application for Therapeutic Abortion Refused

Hans Forssman and Inga Thuwe

INTRODUCTION

The aim of the present study was to determine the mental health, social adjustment and educational level of children born after their mothers had applied for legal abortion on psychiatric grounds, and been refused. For this purpose we compared a series of children born of these pregnancies with an equally large control series, following all the subjects up to their 21st birthday.

Therapeutic abortion was first officially legalized in Sweden in 1939 and during the years of relevance to this study it was permissible on the following grounds (which are still valid):

When, because of disease, physical defect or weakness in the woman, the birth of the child would endanger her life or health.

When the pregnancy is the result of a felony, such as rape or incest, or intercourse with a girl under 15, or of the woman being made to submit to intercourse against her will because of being dependent on the man, or when it is any other way the result of gross violation of the woman's freedom of action.

*Acta Psychiatric Scandinavica, 42:*71-88, 1966

When the expected child might inherit a mental disease, mental deficiency, or a severe physical disease or deformity, either from its mother or father.

On July 1, 1946, the law was broadened to include the following indication:

When, in view of the woman's living conditions or other circumstances, it can be assumed that the birth and care of the expected child will seriously undermine her mental or physical health.

This indication came too late for the mothers of the present subjects. It has led to much debate in Sweden, but the psychiatrists at our hospitals seem to have based their recommendations for or against abortion on essentially the same grounds before 1946 as they did afterwards.

Much has been written about abortion during recent years. Among Swedish studies are: *Lindberg's* (1948) What does the woman do when the psychiatrist says no to her application for abortion?; the social worker *Karin Malmfors'* (1951) follow-up study of 200 women who had applied for abortion; *Ekblad's* follow-up study (1955) of 479 women granted an abortion on psychiatric indications; *Arén & Åmark's* (1957) study of the outcome in 244 cases of authorized but unperformed abortions; *Arén's* (1958) study of 100 newly delivered mothers who had a former pregnancy prematurely terminated on legal grounds; *Kerstin Höök's* (1963) follow-up study of 249 women refused a legal abortion. *Schlaug* (1952) studied the male partner in 488 cases of application for abortion. *Ekblad's* and *Höök's* publications also contained data on the men concerned.

Thus several studies have been made of the mothers and fathers involved in cases of abortion. But little has been written about the third member of the trio involved—the unwanted child. *Arén & Åmark* (1957) related that 12 out of 162 children born to women who had gone through with their pregnancy were sent to a foster home for permanent care or adoption. *Malmfors* (1951) related that 7 out of 85 children born after an application for abortion had been refused were left for adoption. These authors said nothing more about the fate of these children, and *Arén & Åmark* did not check their information in the official registers. Furthermore, both these studies were made between 3 and 5 years after the children were born, when they were too young to permit any conclusion about their mental health or social adjustment. *Höök* (1963) followed a number of features in 204 children in her series until they were 8 1/2 years old, on the average, the ages ranging from 7 to 11 1/2; 15 were left for adoption; the rest of her data about the children cannot be compared with any of the figures from the present study. This seems to be all that is written in Sweden about the fate of these unwanted children.

The Danish author *F. B. Nielsen* (1960), reported that, of 92 children born after application for abortion had been refused, 2 were stillborn, 82 healthy and 8 abnormal in some respect. But his children, too, were too young to permit any conclusion on their mental health and social adjustment.

It is beyond the scope of this investigation to go into the lengthy debate that has been going on about the legislation governing premature termination of pregnancy. Extensive reviews of this are given in the publications of *Ekblad*(1955) and *Höök*(1963).

The problem of abortion was given particular attention in the December 12, 1964, issue of the Lancet, which contained articles by *Tredgold* and by *Uhrus* and a leading article on the subject. The leading article concurred with the demand made at a meeting of U.S.A. specialists in 1955 for "more research into the background, motivation, mechanisms and results" of therapeutic termination of pregnancy.

As therapeutic abortion was not regularized by law in Sweden until January of 1939, it has hardly been possible until now to determine the long-term social and psychiatric consequences for the children born after application for abortion has been refused. In 1960 we published the preliminary results of this study in Swedish.

MATERIAL

Unwanted Children

The subjects studied came from Göteborg, Sweden's second largest city, with a population of about 280,000 at the time in question—1939-1942. During these years, the city had only one large general hospital, the Sahlgren Hospital. In October of 1938, a psychiatric department was opened at the hospital, and among its other activities, this department served as a counselling center for mothers seeking legal abortion. During the years of relevance to the present study, it was the only center of this kind in Göteborg. The few cases taken in hand by private practitioners during this period are not included in our series.

Thus, the material for this investigation originates from all the cases of women living in Göteborg who applied for a therapeutic abortion to the Psychiatric Department of the Sahlgren Hospital during the years 1939 to 1941, inclusive, and were refused. These included both the women coming only to the outpatient service and the ones hospitalized for observation. We took 1941 as the last year so that we could follow the children born of these pregnancies until the age of 21.

During the years 1939 to 1941, altogether 197 women living in Göteborg had 199 applications for legal abortion refused, 2 women having been refused for two pregnancies. These do not include any woman who changed her mind and took back her application. In 188 of the 199, the psychiatrist at the department decided against abortion, in 10 cases, which had been referred to the Medical Board, the Board refused to authorize the abortion, and in one case, also referred to the Medical Board, the Board authorized the abortion but the obstetrician refused to do the operation because the pregnancy had proceeded too far.

Three of the 197 women could not be traced. One was a refugee who lived only a short time in Sweden. It is impossible to explain why the other 2 could not be traced; they may have given a false name or only a temporary address. This left 194 women and 196 refused applications.

Sixty-eight of these 196 pregnancies ended in abortion, spontaneous or provoked. Sixty-eight out of 196 is a large percentage— 34.7 percent—and undoubtedly many of them were illegal. Since the drop-out rate is indicative to some extent of the kind of subjects chosen for study—the narrower the indications for legal abortion, the greater the number of illegal abortions—it is interesting to compare this figure with those from other Nordic countries on the frequency of interrupted pregnancy after legal permission for abortion had been refused. There is not much point in comparing our figures with those of other than these countries because the conditions differ too much.

Lindberg (1948) found that only 50 (14.5 percent) did not give birth at the expected time out of all 344 women refused an authorized abortion after being admitted as inpatients to the Psychiatric Department of the Sahlgren Hospital between 1940 and 1946. *Hultgren*

(1959) found that 14.4 percent of 4,274 women whose petitions for abortion had been turned down by the Medical Board during 1954 to 1956 did not go through with their pregnancy; 224 of the 4,274 were from Göteborg, and 35 of these 224 (15.6 percent) did not go through with their pregnancy.

Thus the percentage of prematurely terminated pregnancies, spontaneous or provoked, was smaller in these two Swedish series than in ours. It is true that all *Lindberg's* women had been under observation as inpatients, as against only 49 of our 199. One probably does not get such a good psychotherapeutic grip on patients only coming to an outpatient service as one does when they are hospitalized. On the other hand, only 83 of 136 Danish women refused legal abortion after observation at the Psychiatric Department at Frederiksberg's Hospital went through with their pregnancies, the drop-out rate in this series thus amounting to 39 percent (*Delcomyn*, 1952).

A more probable explanation for the difference is this. *Lindberg's* series comes from 1940-1946, *Hultgren's* from 1954-1956, and ours from 1939-1941. In 1939 the number of legally authorized abortions in Sweden amounted to 439, in 1946 it rose to 2,378 and in 1951 it reached a peak of 6,328; it then fell slightly, amounting to about 5,000 in 1952-1954, 4,562 in 1955, and 3,851 in 1956. Another way of following the trend is to compare the number of legal abortions with the number of livebirths during the same period. During 1939 to 1942, 0.5 pregnancies were terminated by legal abortion for every hundred livebirths. In 1946 the proportion rose to 1.8, and in 1951 to 5.7. In 1952 and 1954 it was 4.8, in 1955 it was 4.3, and in 1956 it was 3.6.

In short, many more authorized abortions were done after than during the years of relevance to our investigation. Because it was harder to get permission for therapeutic abortion in 1939-1941 than later it is reasonable to assume that more illegal abortions were performed in our series than in later series. *Delcomyn* (1952), comparing the Danish figures for 1945-1949 with those for 1950 and the first half of 1951, found that there were relatively more authorized abortions in the second period, and also that a larger percentage of the women refused a legal abortion went through with their pregnancy the second period. She gave no figures for her observation.

Thus 128 of the pregnancies in our series (representing 126 women) proceeded to term. The result was 134 children, including 6 pairs of twins. Four of the 134 were stillborn, and 8 died within a year, one before it was 2 and one before it was 3. Excluding these 14 cases of early death left 120 children. The present study is based on these 120 all of whom reached the age of 21. They include 4 pairs of twins and 2 twins whose partners had died. Table 1 shows the 120 divided by year of birth and sex.

TABLE 1. *The 120 children born after their mother's application for legal abortion was refused, by year of birth and sex*

Year of birth	Boys	Girls	Total
1939	9	6	15
1940	32	13	45
1941	17	22	39
1942	8	13	21
Total	66	54	120

Control Children

All but 1 of the 120 unwanted children were registered in Göteborg when they were born. We chose control subjects for these 119 as follows: When the infant was born in one of the city's maternity hospitals, we took the next same-sexed child born in the same hospital for its control subject. For the 17 born elsewhere, we took the first same-sexed child registered in the city hospitals on the same day. When the control subject died before the age of 21, we replaced it with the first same-sexed child born after it in the same hospital. For control subjects for twins, we took the next pair of twins, same-sexed or bi-sexed as the case was, born in the same hospital. For the 2 children of twin birth, one of whose partners was stillborn and one died within 3 months, we chose control subjects as if the original children were singletons.

For the control subject of the child born outside Göteborg we took the next child of the same sex registered in the book of the same parish.

SOURCES OF DATA ANALYZED*

From the civil and parish registry offices we found out: whether the would-not-be mother had had her child after her application was turned down; the addresses of the unwanted children and their control subjects from birth until they reached the age of 21; the marital status of the children and whether they in turn had had any children. One control subject lived in another country for six months when she was 18; apart from this we were able to follow every subject from the time they were born until they were 21.

From the child welfare boards (see p. 132) in the various districts in which the subjects had lived, we learned whether they had any of the subject's names in their files and, if so, why.

At the child-guidance clinics and youth psychiatry centers in the districts where the subjects lived or had lived we asked whether they had been consulted for mental deviation or illness in any of the subjects. We did the same at all the mental hospitals and psychiatric departments in general hospitals, and at all the psychiatric outpatient services in the districts where the subjects had lived after the age of 15. We also wrote to all the rural and urban psychiatric consulting bureaus run independently of the psychiatric departments in the general hospitals. We were not able to cover all the private practitioners who might have been consulted and we therefore disregarded anything we happened to hear from one of them having been consulted.

Sweden has a central penal register for the whole country, where every act of the authorities restricting the liberty of an individual is recorded, whether it be sentence to an adult or juvenile prison or internment in some other kind of an institution; also every instance of exemption from legal punishment because of legal irresponsibility, fines above a certain level and fines for crimes for which the alternative is penal servitude. All cases of conditional sentence are also recorded there. After receiving special permission from the government, we went through these files to see whether we could obtain any further evidence of antisocial conduct on the part of the subjects until they reached the age of 21.

*In these analyses we have called a P value of <0.05 probably significant, of <0.01 significant and of <0.001 highly significant.

We also inquired at all the official temperance boards and social agencies in the districts where the subjects lived after the age of 16. (Not until 16 are persons registered in their own names in the records of the social agencies.)

We inquired about the subjects' schooling in the various school districts to which they belonged. Whenever they proceeded to secondary schools, we inquired at these schools whether they had gone on from them to other forms of study, and about any examinations they had passed. Thus we have full information on all the examinations the subjects passed prior to university. We then learned whether they had studied at any university before the age of 21 by going through the annual lists of the students enrolled at the various Swedish universities.

The information we got from the schools and the files of the social agencies showed that there was no point in inquiring at the agencies for the education and care of the mentally retarded.

In Sweden military service is obligatory for men, but not for women. We enquired at the Swedish Institute of Military Psychology about the fitness group into which the male subjects had been classed, and, if they had completed their military service, about how they had succeeded with their duties there. As a rule the young men must enroll for military service the year they become 18, but they can put it off up to the age of 21 or more for reasons of health or education. When they did this, we sometimes extended our limit beyond the 21st birthday in this one respect.

Three subjects (1 original and 2 control subjects) were the children of leading citizens in small communities, and we felt that it would be unfair to make inquiries about them in the local agencies in their neighborhood. But we got all the information we needed about them from other sources and there being no difference between them and the other subjects in depth of penetration we have included them with the others in the various analyses.

DIFFERENCES BETWEEN ORIGINAL AND CONTROL SERIES

Age, Maternal Age and Social Group

The ages of the two series of subjects correspond almost to the day. The greatest difference amounted to 25 days (twin cases).

The unwanted children were born to mothers 30 years old on the average, the control children to mothers of 28, on the average. There is a significant difference here ($0.01 > p > 0.005$).

We also compared the two series for the social group into which they were born, using the norms from the Swedish electoral statistics for the years 1937 to 1940. We did the grouping according to the father's occupation at the time, or if the mother was unmarried according to hers. Children adopted by couples neither of whom was their real parent, were grouped according to the occupation of the adoptive father at the time. But children adopted by men their mothers married after they were born were grouped according to their mothers' occupation when they were born. The result of this comparison is seen from table 2, which also shows how the inhabitants of Göteborg were distributed by social group in 1940.

More of the control than unwanted children were born into group II, and the reverse held for group III. Combining groups I and II gave 25 for the unwanted children and 36 for the control children, against 95 and 84 for group III. Thus the two series did not differ significantly in this respect ($p \simeq 0.10$), though no consideration was given to social group when choosing the control subjects.

Seventy-seven pairs, each consisting of one subject from either series, belonged to the same social group, 43 did not.

TABLE 2. *The unwanted and control children, by original social group*

	Number		Percentage		
Social group	Unwanted children	Control children	Unwanted children	Control children	Whole of Göteborg in 1940
I	3	4	2.5	3.3	6.5
II	22	32	18.3	26.7	31.4
III	95	84	79.2	70.0	62.1
Total	120	120	100.0	100.0	100.0

Results of Comparing Family and Social Environment of Unwanted and Control Children

Insecure Childhood

We considered that the following circumstances in the history of the subjects pointed to an insecure childhood background:

1.   Complaints to a child welfare board about the way the subjects were being treated at home.

Every local authority district in Sweden is required to set up a child welfare board whose duty is to see that all children in its district are properly cared for. Up until 1960 the boards were required to interfere whenever children under 16 were being exposed to physical or mental harm through cruelty or neglect at home, or in danger of becoming delinquent because of their parents' depravity, negligence, or inability to bring up their children.

2.   The child taken into custody by a child welfare board for protective care.

If consulting with, advising or warning the parents had no effect, or if the board decided that it would be a waste of time to try to persuade the parents to mend their ways, the board had the right to take the child away from its parents for protective custody.

3.   Placement in a foster home.

4.   Placement in a children's home.

5.   Childhood in broken home, i.e. loss of a parent through divorce or death before the child was 15, or birth out of wedlock not followed by legitimization.

Table 3 shows how many subjects in either series were brought up under each of these circumstances. As seen there, 32 (26.7 percent) of the unwanted children were born out of wedlock, against only 9 (7.5 percent) of the control children. The difference is highly significant (p <0.001). Eighty-six pairs (one member from each series) agreed in regard to legitimacy; 34 did not. The parents legitimized 5 of the 32 unwanted children born out of wedlock by getting married 2 to 24 months after they were born, and the parents of 5 of the 9 illegitimately born control children did the same 2 to 33 months later. Eight of the unwanted children were adopted by others than their real parents (7 of these were illegitimate). None of the control subjects were adopted.

According to the criteria laid down, 72 (60 percent) of the unwanted children had an insecure childhood, as against only 34 (28.3 percent) of the control children. If one disregards the stays in children's homes, many of which were for only a short while, the figures change to 65 (54.2 percent) against 26 (21.7 percent), and the difference remains highly significant ($p < 0.001$).

In short, it is obvious that the children born after an application for abortion had been refused ran a greater risk of insecurity in childhood than did their control subjects.

TABLE 3. *Comparison between unwanted and control children for circumstances in history pointing to insecurity in childhood (The same child may occur in several categories)*

Circumstances pointing to insecure childhood	Unwanted children	Control children
Report to children's aid bureaus about unsatisfactory conditions at home	17	6
Child removed from home by authorities	2	0
Placement in foster home	19	4
Placement in children's home	30	10
Parents divorced before child was 15	23 ⎫	13 ⎫
Parent(s) died before child was 15	10 ⎬ 60	5 ⎬ 22
Born out of wedlock and never legitimized	27 ⎭	4 ⎭
Born out of wedlock and legitimized	5	5

Disposition to Move to Other Local Authority Districts

There being more delinquency in cities than in other regions we determined how many of either series had stayed the whole time in Göteborg. Another reason for doing so was that we had unusually good possibilities of getting complete information about these subjects since our place of work is in Göteborg. We also checked whether they differed in tendency to move from place to place.

Seventy-seven (62.2 percent) of the unwanted children stayed in Göteborg until they were 21, and 85 (70.8 percent) of the control subjects. Twenty-one (17.5 percent) of the unwanted children had lived in three or more local authority districts, and 19 (15.8 percent) of the control subjects. Thus the two series agreed well, both for permanency of residence in Göteborg, and for tendency to move from one district to another. There were 55 pairs in which both the original and control subject had lived the whole time in Göteborg.

RESULTS OF COMPARING PERSONAL DATA IN ORIGINAL AND CONTROL SERIES

Psychiatric Consultation and Hospitalization

Thirty-four of the unwanted children (28.3 percent) had gone to a psychiatric clinic of some kind or received psychiatric care in a hospital. The corresponding figure for the control subjects was 18, or 15 percent. The difference is probably significant ($0.025 > p > 0.01$).

Twenty-nine of the unwanted children had been under the care of a child psychiatrist, 28 only as an outpatient, and one as an inpatient as well. Six had visited a center for adult psychiatry; 3 of these had been hospitalized, one in a psychiatric department at a general hospital, one at a mental hospital, and one at both. One of the latter belonged to the 29 who had gone to an outpatient department for child and youth psychiatry.

Fifteen of the control subjects had visited a center for child psychiatry, all of them only for outpatient treatment. Four had been patients at a center for adult psychiatry, 2 as an outpatient, one at a mental hospital, and one at both a mental department in a general hospital and a mental hospital. One of these 4 belonged to the 15 who had gone to a center for child psychiatry.

The question arises: Was it because the mothers of the unwanted subjects had been in contact with psychiatrists before the children were born that so many of these children were registered at centers for child psychiatry? It may be that, having once consulted a psychiatrist, these mothers found it easier to do so again, whereas the mothers of the control subjects, who had seldom if ever consulted a psychiatrist about themselves, did not go to a psychiatrist for their children unless something was seriously wrong. Likewise, the mothers who had consulted a psychiatrist about abortion might be more apt than others to seek psychiatric advice for other personal troubles afterwards, and if they then complained about their children being nervous, the child might very likely be sent to a psychiatrist while the perhaps equally nervous children of other mothers might not.

In 1959 we determined how many of the mothers up to that year had consulted a psychiatrist for matters not directly concerned with the abortion, but only among the mothers of the 57 pairs in which both partners had lived in Göteborg all the time up to then. Twenty-seven of the 57 would-not-be mothers had gone to one of the municipal psychiatric outpatient departments for complaints not directly concerned with the abortion, and 10 of their children had done so. The corresponding figures for the control series were 9 and 0. It is apparent from this that it was not because the would-not-be mothers had consulted a psychiatrist about abortion that these children went more often than the others to a child psychiatrist. When all the subjects reached the age of 21, the number of pairs living the whole time in Göteborg dropped to 55, but we did not consider it worth while to do the analysis again for this sake.

Delinquency and Crime

Our figures for acts of delinquent nature reported to the child welfare boards do not cover drunken misconduct; this will be taken up in the next section.

Twenty-two (18.3 percent) of the unwanted subjects, 19 boys and 3 girls, were registered with the child welfare boards for delinquency, against 10 (8.3 percent) of the control subjects, 9 boys and one girl. The difference is probably significant ($p < 0.05$).

The boards had made investigations in 12 of the first 22 subjects and in 4 of the second to determine whether formal charges brought against them should be dropped. This happened 19 times in the original series, 8 times in the control series. Three of the first series and one of the second were removed from their homes and placed in protective custody elsewhere, in accordance with the law then in force, according to which correctional measures must be undertaken when children under 18 show severe forms of maladjustment. One of these 3 unwanted children, as well as the control subject, was sent to a reformatory.

The penal register contained the names of 10 of the unwanted children (8.3 percent) and of 3 control subjects (2.5 percent). The difference is not significant (0.10 >p> 0.05). Nine of the first 10 were male, one was female. The control subjects were all male.

Drunken Misconduct

The records of the official temperance boards contained the names of 19 of the unwanted children (15.8 percent) and 13 control subjects (10.8 percent) for drunken misconduct. The difference is not significant (0.50 >p>0.30). Two of the first 19 subjects were women. The 13 control subjects were all men.

Public Assistance

Seventeen of the unwanted children (14.2 percent) had received some form of public assistance between the ages of 16 and 21, and 3 of the control subjects (2.5 percent). The difference is significant (0.005 >p> 0.001).

Only one subject, a boy in the control series, received a disablement pension from the government; he was an idiot and permanently institutionalized.

Educational Subnormality

Under this heading we included all the uneducable subjects, the ones taught in special schools for the mentally retarded, those whose last year at school was spent in a special class. In the last group we also included a few subjects whose educational subnormality was well documented, but who were taught in ordinary classes because there was no form of special training available for them.

The large cities have a graduated series of special classes in the ordinary schools called remedial reading classes, observation classes, extra classes and health classes, but we paid no attention to the kind of special class the subjects pupil attended, mostly because it depended on where they lived what kind of class they could choose from.

According to these criteria, 13 of the unwanted children (10.8 percent) were educationally subnormal, as against 6 of the control subjects (5.0 percent). This difference is not significant (p = 0.10).

There was one case of well documented mental retardation both in the original and in the control series.

Theoretical Studies Beyond the Obligatory

On drawing a line between the subjects who had done more advanced theoretical study than that required by the school law, and those who had not, we found that only 17 (14.2 percent) of the unwanted had had some form of higher education, as against 40 (33.3 percent) of the control subjects. The difference is highly significant (p < 0.001).

Eight unwanted and 12 control children had taken university entrance examinations. Five unwanted children and 11 control children had studied at a university. Neither of these differences is significant.

As mentioned (table 2), more of the control than original subjects came from social group II and the reverse was true for social group III. As a child's education depends a great deal on the social standing of its parents, we also compared the schooling in the two series after excluding the subjects left over when the two kinds of subjects were paired according to social group. This left 77 subjects in each series. Ten of these 77 (13.0 percent) unwanted children had had some form of higher education, against 21 of the 77 control children (27.3 percent). The difference is probably significant (p < 0.05).

One can also study the effect of social standing on the education by taking one social group at a time; for this we had to combine groups I and II, as there were too few cases in group I. Five of the 95 unwanted children (5.3 percent) coming from group III had had higher education, against 17 of the 84 control subjects (20.2 percent) coming from the same social group. The difference is significant (p < 0.01). The figures for group I + II were 11 out of 25 (44.0 percent) against 28 out of 36 (77.8 percent). Here the difference is probably significant (p <0.05).

Continuing with these calculations, chi square amounts to 7.93 for social group III and to 5.89 for I and II combined. The sum, 13.82, with 2 degrees of freedom gives a p of <0.001, showing a highly significant difference for the three social groups combined.

Thus it was not differences in proportion of different social groups that caused the difference in schooling between the unwanted and control children.

Military Service

Ten of the 66 males in the original series (15.2 percent) were judged unfit for military service, either at the time of enrollment or after they had started, as opposed to 4 (6.7 percent) of the control subjects. This is not a significant difference (0.20 >p> 0.10). According to our information, 4 of the 10 first males were exempted for mental reasons; our information in this respect may not be complete, however. Two of the control subjects were exempted on these grounds.

When a Swedish recruit enrolls, he is classified into one of four groups according to his fitness for military service, from group 1 for a completely satisfactory condition down to group 4 who are assigned to fatigue duty. Apart from exemption from service, our two series were distributed very much alike by fitness for military service.

Marital Status and Parenthood

As we only followed our subjects up to the age of 21, we cannot say much about how they compare with regard to marriage and parenthood. Some differences did emerge, however.

Twenty of the unwanted children (17 women, 3 men) married before the age of 21, and 14 of the control subjects (9 women, 5 men). The difference is not significant here, either for the sexes combined or for one of them.

Two of the female subjects from the original series had also divorced before the age of 21; none of the control women had done so, and no man from either series.

We restricted our analysis of parenthood to the women, as there was no hope of getting reliable figures for the men in this respect.

Fourteen out of 54 women from the original series had had 19 children before they were 21, 4 out of wedlock, and 7 of the 54 female control subjects had had 9 children, 3 out of wedlock.

It is impossible to draw any conclusions from these figures. It will be noted, however, that the control series (which had more education on the whole) contained fewer cases of early marriage and of young mothers. This tallies with the observation that the age of marriage and parenthood rise with the degree of education.

Freedom From Defect in All Respects Studied

Sometimes the same subject will occur in more than one of the groups studied here. Thus a subject registered with the authorities for abuse of alcohol will often be found in the files of the centers for child psychiatry as well; a man who has been in a mental hospital will sometimes be exempted from military service; an uneducable subject will be registered as receiving public assistance, as being educated in a special class, and so on. It is interesting, therefore, to compare the two series for the number of subjects showing no defect in any of the respects studies, i.e., registration for antisocial behavior in the books of the child welfare boards or penal register; official registration for drunken misconduct; education in a special class or school, or uneducability; public assistance or government pension; visits to psychiatric inpatient or outpatient departments during childhood or adulthood. Fifty-eight (48.3 percent) of the unwanted children showed none of these defects against 82 (68.3 percent) of the control subjects. The difference is significant (0.005 >p> 0.001).

Taking social group III separately from I and II combined showed the following: Forty of the 95 unwanted children (42.1 percent) coming from group III showed no defect, against 54 of the 84 control subjects (64.3 percent) from the same group. The difference is significant (0.005 >p> 0.001). The corresponding figures for group I and II combined were 19 out of 25 (76.0 percent) against 28 out of 36 (77.8 percent). Here the difference is not significant.

The same analysis of the 77 pairs concordant for social group gave 34 unwanted cases (44.2 percent) showing no defect, against 54 control (70.1 percent). The difference is significant (0.005 >p> 0.001).

Similar analysis of the 55 pairs living in Göteborg the whole time gave 20 (36.4 percent) showing no defect against 38 (69.1 percent). The difference is highly significant (p <0.001).

As children from broken homes are more apt than others to be antisocial and mentally disturbed, we compared the two series for the number of cases showing none of the aforementioned defects among the subjects who had lived with both their real parents until they were 15. Thirty-three out of the 60 such subjects from the original series (55.0 percent) showed none of these defects, and 68 out of the 98 control subjects of this category (69.4 percent). The difference is not significant (0.10 >p> 0.05).

DISCUSSION

Table 4 gives a survey of the ways in which the children born after their mother had been refused a legal abortion differed from the control series of same-aged subjects chosen at random. As seen there, the unwanted children were worse off in every respect, the only exception being due to the one case of a government pension which came from the control series. The differences were often significant, and when they were not, they pointed in the same direction (except for the case just mentioned)—to a worse lot for the unwanted children.

When one looks for a reason for the differences, one is struck mostly by the greater frequency of factors tending to disrupt the stability of the home in the case of the unwanted children, such as birth out of wedlock, and death or divorce of their parents while they were still young. In other words, not as many unwanted children were brought up by both their real parents as were control subjects. Probably as a corollary of this, more of them were brought up by foster parents of in children's homes. But the latter may also have been a consequence of the greater number of complaints to the children's welfare boards about the way in which they were being treated at home.

The difference that turned up most consistently in various forms of analysis was the difference in amount of education. Whatever categories of subjects were studied—different social ranks or different subgroups of the same social rank—the unwanted children got a significantly smaller amount of education than the control subjects.

The reason the unwanted children had had so much contact with psychiatrists was probably not—as we showed—that their mothers

TABLE 4. *Survey of important differences between the unwanted and control children*

	Unwanted children			Control children			Level of sign. of differ.
	No. in resp. series	Feature present		No. in resp. series	Feature present		
		No.	%		No.	%	
Psychiatric consultation and hospitalization	120	34	28.3	120	18	15.0	*
Registration for delinquency at children's aid bureaus	120	22	18.3	120	10	8.3	*
Registration for crime in Penal Register	120	10	8.3	120	3	2.5	—
Registration for drunken misconduct	120	19	15.8	120	13	10.8	—
Public assistance between age of 16 and 21	120	17	14.2	120	3	2.5	**
Subnormal educability or uneducability	120	13	10.8	120	6	5.0	—
Theoretical studies beyond the obligatory:							
Whole series	120	17	14.2	120	40	33.3	***
Subjects in pairs congruent for social group	77	10	13.0	77	21	27.3	*
Subjects from social group III	95	5	5.3	84	17	20.2	**
Subjects from social groups I + II	25	11	44.0	36	28	77.8	*
Exemption from military service	66	10	15.2	66	4	6.7	—
Freedom from inferiority in above respects:							
Whole series	120	58	48.3	120	82	68.3	**
Social group III	95	40	42.1	84	54	64.3	**
Social groups I + II	25	19	76.0	36	28	77.8	—

Subjects in pairs congruent for social group	77	34	44.2	77	54	70.1	**
Subjects living all their life in Göteborg	55	20	36.4	55	38	69.1	***
Subjects brought up by both their real parents	60	33	55.0	98	68	69.4	—

found it easier to consult a psychiatrist about their child because they had once before consulted a psychiatrist about themselves. It was probably because these mothers were more vulnerable mentally than the others, and passed on this failing to their children, either through genes or through the effect it had on the home environment, or both.

The investigation has shown that children born after their mothers have been refused permission for legal abortion are born into a worse situation than other children. From this one may assume that the children who are not born because their mothers get authorization for abortion would have had to face still greater disadvantages, socially and mentally. Thus, the very fact that a woman seeks an authorized abortion, no matter how trivial her grounds may appear to some, means that the expected child will run a larger risk than its peers of an inferior standing in life. In our opinion, the present investigation shows that the provisions for therapeutic abortion in the law should not only aim to prevent the private tragedy; they should also aim to improve mental hygiene in a wider sense. Thus the legislation should also consider the social handicaps awaiting the unwanted child, not only, as it does now, the genetic risk in the narrow sense of the terms.

SUMMARY

The authors examined 120 children born after their mothers had applied for therapeutic abortion on psychiatric grounds and been refused, comparing them with an appropriate control series of the same size. All the subjects studied lived and were followed up until the age of 21. Data were assembled from civil and ecclesiastical registry offices, social agencies, school authorities, military authorities and all the psychiatric inpatient and outpatient departments everywhere the subjects had lived. It was ascertained how many of each series had been registered for mental ill-health, antisocial and criminal actions, drunken misconduct, and different forms of public assistance; for the men it was ascertained how they had got on during their military service; likewise the marital status, number of children, and school ability and educational level was determined.

A study of the social features revealed that many more of the unwanted than control children had not had the advantage of a secure family life during childhood. They were also registered more often in psychiatric services, and a few more of them than control subjects received psychiatric care. They were more often registered for antisocial and criminal behavior, and slightly more often for drunken misconduct, and they got public assistance more often than the control subjects. A few more of them were educationally subnormal and far fewer had pursued theoretical studies over and above what is obligatory. They were more often exempted from military service. More of the females married early and had children early than in the control series. The differences between the two series in these respects were often statistically significant, and when they were not significant they always pointed in the same direction—to the unwanted children being born into a worse situation than the control children. Table 4 gives figures for most of the features just mentioned.

The authors conclude that the very fact a woman applies for legal abortion means that the prospective child runs a risk of having to surmount greater social and mental handicaps than its peers, even when the grounds for the application are so slight that it is refused. In their opinion, the legislation of therapeutic termination of pregnancy should also consider the social risks to which the expected child will be exposed.

REFERENCES

Arén, P. (1958): Undersökning av 100 nyblivna mödrar med legal abort i anamnesen (One hundred newly delivered mothers with a history of legal abortion). *Svenska Läk.-Tidn.* 55, 505-522.

Arén, P., & C. Åmark (1957): Prognosen vid beviljad men icke utförd legal abort (Outcome in cases of authorized but not performed therapeutic abortion). *Svenska Läk.-Tidn.* 54, 3709-3784.

Delcomyn, K. (1952): Efterundersogelse af Kvinder, der har fået Afslag på Anmodning om Abortus provocatus (Follow-up study of women whose application for therapeutic abortion was refused). *Nord. Med. 48,* 980.

Ekblad, M. (1955): Induced abortion on psychiatric grounds. *Acta psychiat. scand.,* supp. 99.

Forssman, H., & I. Thuwe (1960): En socialpsykiatrisk efterundersökning av 120 barn födda efter avslag på abortframställning (Mental health and social adjustment of 120 children born after application for therapeutic abortion refused). *Nord. psykiat. T. 14,* 265-279.

Hultgren, G. (1959): Avslag på ansökan om legal abort (Application for legal abortion refused). *Nord. Med. 62,* 1182-1185.

Höök, K. (1963): Refused abortion. A follow-up study of 249 women whose applications were refused by the National Board of Health in Sweden. *Acta psychiat. scand.,* supp. 168.

Lancet (1964): Termination of pregnancy on psychiatric grounds, Leading article in II, Dec. 12.

Lindberg, B. F. (1948): Vad gör den abortsökande kvinnan när psykiatern sagt nej? (What does the woman do when the psychiatrist says no to her application for abortion?). *Svenska Läk.-Tidn. 45,* 1381-1391.

Malmfors, K. (1951): Den abortsökande kvinnans problem (Problems of the woman seeking abortion). *Svenska Läk.-Tidn 48,* 2445-2468.

Nielsen, F. B. (1960): Afgorelser i et Modrehjelpssamråd og en Efterundersogelse (Decisions by a maternity assistance board and a follow-up study). *Ugeskr. Laeg. 120,* 330-335.

Schlaug, R. (1952): Om de abortsökande kvinnoras män (The male partners of women applying for therapeutic abortion). *Svenska Läk.-Tidn. 49,* 849-862.

Svensk författningssamling (Swedish Statue Code) (1938): Lag om avbrytande av havandeskap (Legislation on abortion). No. 318, Stockholm.

Sveriges officiella statistik (Official Swedish statistics) (1941): Riksdagsmannavalen åren 1937-1940 (Government election statistics for 1937-1941). Stockholm.

Sveriges officiella statistik (Official Swedish statistics) (1959): Allmän hälso- och sjukwärd 1957 (Public health and care of the sick in 1957). Stockholm.

Text till lag om samhällets barnavärd och ungdomsskydd (Proposed wording for the legislation governing official supervision of child welfare and protection of youth) (1950): Svenska social-värdsförbundet (Swedish Social Welfare Association), Stockholm.

Tredgold, R. F. (1964): Psychiatric indications for termination of pregnancy. *Lancet*, 12 Dec., *7372*, 1251-1254.

Uhrus, K. (1964): Some aspects of the Swedish law governing termination of pregnancy. *Lancet*, 12 Dec. *7372*, 1292-1293.

The People, Plaintiff & Respondent
v.
Leon Phillip Belous Defendent & Appellant

PETERS, Justice.

Dr. Leon Phillip Belous was convicted in January 1967, after a jury trial, of abortion, in violation of section 274 of the Penal Code, and conspiracy to commit an abortion, in violation of section 182 of the Penal Code, both felonies. The court suspended proceedings, imposed a fine of $5,000, and placed Dr. Belous on probation for two years. He appeals from the order granting probation.

Dr. Belous is a physician and surgeon, licensed since 1931 to practice medicine in the State of California, and specializing in obstetrics and gynecology. He has been on the attending staff of the gynecology department of Cedars of Lebanon Hospital in Los Angeles since 1931, is a fellow of the Los Angeles Gynecology and Obstetrical Society, the American College of Obstetrics and Gynecology, The Abdominal Surgical Society, and the Geriatric Society, and a member of the American Board of Obstetrics and Gynecology. He is on the Board of Directors of the California Committee on Therapeutic

Supreme Court of California, In Bank. Sept. 5, 1969. Rehearing Denied October 1, 1969. Cr. 12739 71 Cal. 2d 996, 458 P. 2d 194, 80 Cal. Rptr. 354 (1969)

Abortion, an organization which seeks to liberalize abortion laws. He is considered by his associates to be an eminent physician in his field.

The prosecution's witnesses, a young woman and her husband, Cheryl and Clifton, testified to the following:

In 1966, Cheryl, then unmarried, believed she was pregnant. A family physician had given her pills which would induce menstruation if she were not pregnant, but the pills did not work. She and Clifton had sometime earlier seen Dr. Belous on television, advocating a change in the California abortion laws. They had never heard of Dr. Belous before. Clifton obtained the doctor's phone number from the television station and phoned Dr. Belous; he explained the problem and that they both were "pretty disturbed," and at their "wit's end" and asked for Dr. Belous' help. Dr. Belous told him there was nothing he could do, but Clifton "continued pleading," and threatened that Cheryl would go to Tijuana for an abortion. Finally the doctor agreed to see them at his office.

Dr. Belous examined Cheryl at his Beverly Hills office and confirmed that she was possibly pregnant. Cheryl was otherwise in good health. The visit lasted about 45 minutes and was very emotional. Both Clifton and Cheryl pleaded for help, cried, insisted they were going to have an abortion "one way or another." The doctor lectured them on the dangers of criminal abortions, and Tijuana abortions in particular, and suggested that they get married. He insisted he did not perform abortions. He refused to recommend anyone in Tijuana. Finally, in response to their pleadings, Dr. Belous gave them a piece of paper with a Chula Vista phone number. He told them an abortion would cost about $500. He gave Cheryl a prescription for some antibiotics and instructed her to return for an examination.

Dr. Belous testified that he was very familiar with the abortion business in Tijuana. He had visited clinics there to learn about conditions and knew that women who went to Tijuana were taking their lives in their hands. He met Karl Lairtus while in Tijuana and knew from personal observation that Lairtus, licensed to practice in Mexico but not in California, was performing skilled and safe abortions in Mexico. Lairtus wanted to obtain a California license, and sought out Belous' help on a number of occasions. When Lairtus moved from Mexico to Chula Vista, he gave Dr. Belous his address and phone number. When Lairtus moved to Los Angeles, he gave the doctor a

Hollywood address, and made it known to the doctor that he was performing abortions. It was Lairtus' number that Belous gave to Cheryl and Clifton. Although he had given out Lairtus' number before, in similar situations, where distraught pregnant women insisted they would do anything, Dr. Belous had no idea how many women actually went to Lairtus.

Cheryl and Clifton made arrangements with Lairtus, and went to the address which Lairtus gave them on the phone. After the abortion was performed, while Cheryl was resting, the police, having been advised by another woman that Lairtus was performing abortions at that address, came to his apartment, followed another couple into the apartment and arrested Lairtus. They found two notebooks containing women's names, ages, dates of last menstruation, and physician's names, including Dr. Belous' name, which the police interpreted as the referring doctor with whom Lairtus was to split his fees. On the basis of this information, Dr. Belous was arrested at his office. Lairtus pleaded guilty. At Dr. Belous' trial, he testified that, although not solicited, he sent Dr. Belous about $100 as a professional courtesy in about half the cases that he had performed abortions on Dr. Belous' patients. Dr. Belous denied receiving any money from Lairtus.

The substance of Dr. Belous' defense was that he gave Lairtus' phone number to Cheryl and Clifton only because he believed that they would, in fact, do anything to terminate the pregnancy, which might involve butchery in Tijuana or self-mutilation; that in face of their pleading and tears, he gave out the phone number of someone whom he knew to be a competent doctor, although unlicensed in this state. The doctor believed that if the young couple carried out their threats, Cheryl's very life was in danger.

Section 274 of the Penal Code, when the conduct herein involved occurred, read: "Every person who provides, supplies, or administers to any woman, or procures any woman to take any medicine, drug, or substance, or uses or employs any instrument or other means whatever, with intent thereby to procure the miscarrage of such woman, unless the same is necessary to preserve her life, is punishable by imprisonment in the State prison not less than two nor more than five years."

The statute was substantially unchanged since it was originally enacted in 1850(1). In 1967, the statute was amended and sections 25950 through 25954 *(Therapeutic Abortion Act)* added to the

Health and Safety Code. The act extends the lawful grounds for obtaining an abortion(2). Section 274 is directed towards the abortionist. Under section 275 of the Penal Code (also amended by the *Therapeutic Abortion Act*), a woman who solicits or submits to an abortion is punishable by up to five years' imprisonment; similarly, under section 276, any person who solicits a woman to submit to an abortion is punishable by up to five years' imprisonment.

We have concluded that the term "necessary to preserve" in section 274 of the Penal Code is not susceptible of a construction that does not violate legislative intent and that is sufficiently certain to satisfy due process requirements without improperly infringing on fundamental constitutional rights.

"The requirement of a reasonable degree of certainty in legislation, especially in the criminal law, is a well established element of the guarantee of due process of law. 'No one may be required at peril of life, liberty or property to speculate as to the meaning of penal statutes. All are entitled to be informed as to what the State commands or forbids. . . . "A statute which either forbids or requires the doing of an act in terms so vague that men of common intelligence must necessarily guess at its meaning and differ as to its application, violates the first essential of due process of law." ' *Lanzetta v. New Jersey,* 306 U.S. 451, 453, 59 S.Ct. 618, 83 L.Ed. 888; see also *Connally v. General Const. Co.,* 269 U.S. 385, 391, 46 S.Ct. 126, 70 L.Ed. 322. Such also is the law of the State of California. *People v. McCaughan,* 49 Cal.2d 409, 414, 317 P.2d 974.

1.   "The required meaning, certainty and lack of ambiguity may appear on the face of the questioned statute or from any demonstrably established technical or common law meaning of the language in question. *People v. McCaughan, supra,* 49 Cal. 2d 409, 414, 317 P.2d 974; *Lorenson v. Superior Court,* 35 Cal.2d 49, 60, 216 P.2d 859." (In re Newbern, 53 Cal.2d 786, 792, 3 Cal.Rptr. 364, 368, 350 P.2d 116, 120.) The requirement of certainty in legislation is greater where the criminal statute is a limitation on constitutional rights. (See *Smith v. California* (1959) 361 U.S. 147, 151, 80 S.Ct. 215, 4 L.Ed.2d 205.) On the other hand, mathematical certainty is not required; "some matter of degree" is involved in most penal statutes. *(Nash v. United States* (1913) 229 U.S. 373, 377, 33 S.Ct. 780, 57 L.Ed. 1232.)

Dictionary definitions and judicial interpretations fail to provide a clear meaning for the words, "necessary" or "preserve." There is, of course, no standard definition of "necessary to preserve," and taking the words separately, no clear meaning emerges. "Necessary" is defined as: "1) Essential to a desirable or projected end or condition; not to be dispensed with without loss, damage, inefficiency, or the like; . . . " (Webster's New International Dictionary (2d ed.), unabridged.) The courts have recognized that " 'necessary' has not a fixed meaning, but is flexible and relative." *(Westphal v. Westphal,* 122 Cal. App. 379, 382, 10 P.2d 119, 120; see also, *City of Dayton v. Borchers* (Ohio Common Pleas, 1967) 13 Ohio Misc. 273, 232 N.E.2d 437, 441 ["A *necessary* thing may supply a wide range of wants, from mere convenience to logical completeness."].)

The definition of "preserve" is even less enlightening. It is defined as: "1) To keep or save from injury or destruction; to guard or defend from evil; to protect; save. 2) To keep in existence or intact; . . . To save from decomposition, . . . 3) To maintain; to keep up; . . . (Webster's New International Dictionary, *supra.*) The meanings for "preserve" range from the concept of maintaining the status quo—that is, the women's condition of life at the time of pregnancy—to maintaining the biological or medical definition of "life"—that is, as opposed to the biological or medical definition of "death."

Since abortion before quickening was not a crime at common law (Perkins, Criminal Law (1957) 101; Means, The Law of New York Concerning Abortion and the Status of the Fetus, 1664-1968: A Case of Cessation of Constitutionality (1968) 14 N.Y.L. F. 411, 419-422; Stern, Abortion: Reform and the Law (1968) 59 J.Crim.L.C. & P.S. 84, 85) we cannot rely on common law meanings or common law referents (see *Lorenson v. Superior Court, supra,* 35 Cal. 2d 49, 60, 216 P.2d 859; *People v. Agnello,* 259 Cal.App.2d 785, 790-791, 66 Cal.Rptr. 571)(3).

Various possible meanings of "necessary to preserve . . . life" have been suggested. However, none of the proposed definitions will sustain the statute.

Respondent asserts: "If medical science feels the abortion should be performed as it is necessary to preserve her life, then it may be performed; that is, unless it is performed the patient will die."

Our courts, however, have rejected an interpretation of "necessary to preserve" which requires certainty or immediacy of death. *(People v. Abarbanel,* 239 Cal.App. 2d 31, 32, 35, 48 Cal.Rptr. 336; *People v. Ballard,* 218 Cal.App.2d 295, 298, 32 Cal. Rptr. 233; *People v. Ballard,*

167 Cal.App. 2d 803, 807, 335 P.2d 204.) Justice Fourt, in *People v. Ballard, supra,* 167 Cal.App. 2d 803, 814, 335 P.2d 204, 212, stated: "Surely, the abortion statute (Pen.Code, § 274) does not mean by the words 'unless the same is necessary to preserve her life' that the peril to life be imminent. It ought to be enough that the dangerous condition 'be potentially present, even though its full development might be delayed to a greater or less extent. Nor was it essential that the doctor should believe that the death of the patient would be otherwise *certain* in order to justify him in affording present relief.' [Citations.]" The above language was quoted in *People v. Abarbanel, supra,* 239 Cal.App.2d 31, 34, 48 Cal.Rptr. 336.

In *People v. Ballard, supra,* 167 Cal.App. 2d 803, 813-814, 335 P.2d 204, 211, the evidence established that the woman was "extremely nervous . . . upset, had headaches, was unable to sleep, and thought that she was pregnant. She was agitated, disturbed and had many problems." (Italics omitted.) In *People v. Ballard, supra,* 218 Cal.App.2d 295, 307, 32 Cal.Rptr. 233, it was established that at the time each of the women went to the defendant doctor she was in a "bad state of health" because of self-imposed abortive practices. And in *People v. Abarbanel, supra,* 239 Cal.App.2d 31, 48 Cal.Rptr. 336, the obstetrician performed the abortion after receiving letters from two psychiatrists to the effect that abortion was indicated as necessary to save the woman's life from the "possibility" of suicide. In each of the cases the conviction was reversed.

If the fact of ill health or the mere "possibility" of suicide is sufficient to meet the test of "necessary to preserve her life," it is clear that a showing of immediacy or certainty of death is not essential for a lawful abortion. Two other jurisdictions have also rejected an interpretation of "necessary to preserve" which would require certainty or immediacy of death. *(State v. Dunklebarger* (1928) 206 Iowa 971, 221 N. W. 592, 596; *State v. Hatch* (1917), 138 Minn. 317, 164 N.W. 1017.)

After the decision in *Ballard,* the Legislature did not amend the statute to repudiate the rule suggested by that case and to establish a definition requiring certainty of death(4).

It would be anomalous to uphold a criminal statute against a charge of vagueness by adopting a construction of the statute rejected by the courts of this state as not reflecting legislative intent unless there was a clear showing of a strong public policy or legislative intent requiring adoption of the rejected construction. No such showing has been made with regard to the construction urged by respondent.

Moreover, a definition requiring certainty of death would work an invalid abridgment of the woman's constitutional rights. The rights involved in the instant case are the woman's rights to life and to choose whether to bear children(5). The woman's right to life is involved because childbirth involves risks of death(6).

2 & 3.   The fundamental right of the woman to choose whether to bear children follows from the Supreme Court's and this court's repeated acknowledgment of a "right of privacy" or "liberty" in matters related to marriage, family, and sex. (See, e.g., *Griswold v. Connecticut, supra,* 381 U.S. 479, 485, 486, 500, 85 S.Ct. 1678, 14 L.Ed.2d 510; *Loving v. Virginia* (1967) 388 U.S. 1, 12, 87 S.Ct. 1817, 18 L.Ed.2d 1010 [statute prohibiting interracial marriages, violative of Due Process Clause]; *Skinner v. Oklahoma ex rel. Williamson* (1942) 316 U.S. 535, 536, 541, 62 S.Ct. 1110, 86 L.Ed. 1655 [sterilization laws; marriage and procreation involve a "basic liberty"]; *Pierce v. Society of Sisters* (1925) 268 U.S. 510, 534-535, 45 S.Ct. 571, 69 L.Ed. 1070, 39 A.L.R. 468 [prohibition against nonpublic schools; same]; *Meyer v. Nebraska* (1923) 262 U.S. 390, 399-400, 43 S.Ct. 625, 67 L.Ed. 1042 [prohibition against teaching children German language; same]; *Perez v. Sharp,* 32 Cal.2d 711, 715, 198 P.2d 17; see also *Custodio v. Bauer,* 251 Cal.App.2d 303, 317-318, 59 Cal.Rptr. 463.) That such a right is not enumerated in either the United States or California Constitutions is not impediment to the existence of the right. (See, e.g., *Carrington v. Rash* (1965) 380 U.S. 89, 96, 85 S.Ct. 775, 13 L.Ed.2d 675 [fundamental but nonenumerated right to vote]; *Aptheker v. Secretary of State* (1964) 378 U.S. 500, 505-506, 84 S.Ct. 1659, 12 L.Ed.2d 992 and *Kent v. Dulles* (1958) 357 U.S. 116, 125, 78 S.Ct. 1113, 2 L.Ed.2d 1204 [right to travel]; *Bolling v. Sharpe* (1954) 347 U.S. 497, 500, 74 S.Ct. 693, 98 L.Ed. 884 [right to attend federal unsegregated schools]; *Otsuka v. Hite,* 64 Cal.2d 596, 602, 51 Cal.Rptr. 284, 414 P.2d 412 [right to vote]; cf. *Finot v. Pasadena City Bd. of Education,* 250 Cal. App.2d 189, 199, 58 Cal.Rptr. 520.) It is not surprising that none of the parties who have filed briefs in this case have disputed the existence of this fundamental right.

The critical issue is not whether such rights exist, but whether the state has a compelling interest in the regulation of a subject which is within the police powers of the state *(Shapiro v. Thompson* (1969), 394

U.S. 618, 89 S.Ct. 1322, 22 L.Ed.2d 600; *Sherbert v. Verner* (1963) 374 U.S. 398, 403, 83 S.Ct. 1790, 10 L.Ed.2d 965), whether the regulation is "necessary . . . to the accomplishment of a permissible state policy" *(McLaughlin v. Florida* (1964) 379 U.S. 184, 196, 85 S.Ct. 283, 290, 13 L.Ed.2d 222; see also, *N.A.A.C.P. v. Button,* 371 U.S. 415, 438, 83 S.Ct. 328, 9 L.Ed.2d 405; *Bates v. City of Little Rock* (1960) 361 U.S. 516, 527, 80 S.Ct. 412, 4 L.Ed.2d 480; *Huntley v. Public Util. Comm.,* 69 A.C. 62, 69, 69 Cal.Rptr. 605, 442 P.2d 685; *Vogel v. County of Los Angeles,* 68 Cal.2d 18, 21, 64 Cal.Rptr. 409, 434 P.2d 961; *People v. Woody,* 61 Cal.2d 716, 718, 40 Cal.Rptr. 69, 394 P.2d 813), and whether legislation impinging on constitutionally protected areas is narrowly drawn and not of "unlimited and indiscriminate sweep" *(Shelton v. Tucker* (1960) 364 U.S. 479, 490, 81 S.Ct. 247, 5 L.Ed.2d 231; see also, *Cantwell v. Connecticut* (1940) 310 U.S. 296, 308, 60 S.Ct. 900, 84 L.Ed. 1213; In re Berry, 68 Cal.2d 137, 151, 65 Cal.Rptr. 273, 436 P.2d 273; In re Hoffman, 67 Cal.2d 845, 853-854, 64 Cal.Rptr. 97, 434 P.2d 353).

It is possible that the definition suggested by respondent, requiring that death be certain, was that intended by the Legislature when the first abortion law was adopted in 1850 and that, in the light of the then existing medical and surgical science, the great and direct interference with a woman's constitutional rights was warranted by considerations of the woman's health. When California's first anti-abortion statute was enacted, any surgical procedure which entered a body cavity was extremely dangerous. Surgeons did not know how to control infection, and mortality was high. (Haagensen & Lloyd, A Hundred Years of Medicine (1943) p. 19.) In 1867, Joseph Lister first published his findings on antiseptic surgery *(id.,* at pp. 241-242), but even in 1883 the techniques he developed were condemned *(id.,* at p. 245), and as late as 1895 were not well understood or properly applied by even leaders of the medical profession. *(Id.,* at p. 246; see also, H. Robb (1895) Aseptic Surgical Technique.)

Although development was slow, techniques of antisepsis and asepsis became major general advances in surgery at and after the turn of the century. In due course safe procedures were developed for specific operations. Curettage, used for abortion in the first trimester, became a safe, accepted and routinely employed medical technique, especially after antibiotics were developed in the early 1940's. (Douglas, Toxic Effects of the Welch Bacillus in Postabortal Infections (1956) 56

N.Y.State J.Med. 3673.) It is now safer for a woman to have a hospital therapeutic abortion during the first trimester than to bear a child(7).

Although abortions early in pregnancy and properly performed present minimal danger to the woman, criminal(8) abortions are "the most common single cause of maternal deaths in California." (Fox, Abortion Deaths in California (1967) 98 Am.J.Obst. & Gynec. 645, 650.) In California, it is estimated that 35,000 to 100,000 such abortions occur each year. (Fox, *supra,* at p. 645.)

The incidence of severe infection from criminal abortion is very much greater than the incidence of death. The Los Angeles County Hospital alone, for example, in 1961 admitted over 3,500 patients treated for such abortions. (Kistner, Medical Indications for Contraception: Changing Viewpoints (editorial) (1965) 25 Obst. & Gynec. 285, 286.) Possibly more significant than the mere incidence of infection caused by criminal abortions is the result of such infection. "Induced Illegal Abortion . . . is one of the important causes of subsequent infertility and pelvic disease." (Kleegman & Kaufman, Infertility in Women (1966) p. 301; see also Curtis & Huffman, Gynecology (6th ed. 1950) pp. 564-566)(9).

Amici for appellant, 178 deans of medical schools, including the deans of all California medical schools, chairmen of medical school departments, and professors of medical school departments, and professors of medical schools state: "These recorded facts bring one face-to-face with the hard, shocking—almost brutal—reality that our statute designed in 1850 to protect women from serious risks to life and health has in modern times becomes a scourge"(10).

Constitutional concepts are not static. Our United States Supreme Court said, regarding the equal protection clause of the Fourteenth Amendment: "We agree, of course, with Mr. Justice Holmes that the Due Process Clause of the Fourteenth Amendment 'does not enact Mr. Herbert Spencer's Social Statics.' [Citation.] Likewise, the Equal Protection Clause is not shackled to the political theory of a particular era. In determining what lines are unconstitutionally discriminatory, we have never been confined to historic notions of equality, any more than we have restricted due process to a fixed catalogue of what was at a given time deemed to be authorized to practice surgery, carried out the limits of fundamental rights. . . . *(Harper v. Virginia State Bd. of Elections* (1966) 383 U.S. 663, 669, 86 S.Ct. 1079, 1082, 16 L.Ed.2d 169; see also, *Perez v. Sharp, supra,*

32 Cal.2d 711, 727, 198 P.2d 17; *Galyon v. Municipal Court,* 229 Cal. App.2d 667, 671-672, 40 Cal.Rptr. 446, and cases cited therein ["[A] statute valid when enacted may become invalid by change in the conditions to which it is applied."]. See also, Means, *supra,* 14 N.Y.L.F. 411, 514-515.)

In the light of modern medical surgical practice, the great and direct infringement of constitutional rights which would result from a definition requiring certainty of death may not be justified on the basis of considerations of the woman's health where, as here, abortion is sought during the first trimester.

It is next urged that the state has a compelling interest in the protection of the embryo and fetus(11) and that such interest warrants the limitation on the woman's constitutional rights. Reliance is placed upon several statutes and court rules which assertedly show that the embryo or fetus is equivalent to a born child. However, all of the statutes and rules relied upon require a live birth or reflect the interest of the parents(12).

In any event, there are major and decisive areas where the embryo and fetus are not treated as equivalent to the born child. Probably the most important is reflected by the statute before us. The intentional destruction of the born child is murder or manslaughter. The intentional destruction of the embryo or fetus is never treated as murder, and only rarely as manslaughter but rather as the lesser offense of abortion. (Perkins, Criminal Law, *supra,* p. 103; Means, *supra,* 14 N.Y.L.F. at p. 445)(13).

Furthermore, the law has always recognized that the pregnant woman's right to life takes precedence over any interest the state may have in the unborn. The California abortion statutes, as to the abortion laws of all 51 United States jurisdictions, make an exception in favor of the life of the prospective mother. (See Stern, Abortion: Reform and the Law, *supra,* 59 J. Crim.L.C. & P.S. 84, 86-87; George, Current Abortion Laws: Proposals & Movements for Reform (1965) 17 W.Res.L.Rev. 366, 375.) Although there may be doubts as to whether the state's interest may ever justify requiring a woman to risk death, it is clear that the state could not forbid a woman to procure an abortion where, to a medical certainty, the result of childbirth would be death. We are also satisfied that the state may not require that degree of risk involved in respondent's definition, which would prohibit an abortion, where death from childbirth although not medically certain, would be substantially certain or more likely than not. Accordingly, the definition of the statute suggested by respondent must be rejected as an invalid infringement upon the woman's constitutional rights.

4. Although we may assume that the law was valid when first enacted, the validity of a law in 1850 does not resolve the issue of whether the law is constitutionally valid today. (Compare, e.g., *Gray v. Sanders* (1963) 372 U.S. 368, 381, 83 S.Ct. 801, 9 L.Ed.2d 821, with *South v. Peters* (1950) 339 U.S. 276, 277, 70 S.Ct. 641, 94 L.Ed. 834; *Baker v. Carr* (1962) 369 U.S. 186, 237, 82 S.Ct. 691, 7 L.Ed.2d 663, with *Colegrove v. Green* (1946) 328 U.S. 549, 556, 66 S.Ct. 1198, 90 L.Ed. 1432; *Brown v. Board of Education* (1954) 347 U.S. 483, 495, 74 S.Ct. 686, 98 L.Ed. 873; with *Plessy v. Ferguson* (1896) 163 U.S. 537, 550-551, 16 S.Ct. 1138, 41 L.Ed. 256.)

Another definition of the term "necessary to preserve" is suggested by *People v. Abarbanel, supra,* 239 Cal.App.2d 31, 32, 34, 48 Cal.Rptr. 336, where the court held that an abortion was not unlawful where the obstetrician performed the abortion based on the "possibility" of suicide. *Abarbanel* might be understood as meaning that "necessary to preserve" refers to a possibility of death different from or greater than the ordinary risk of childbirth. To so interpret "necessary to preserve" would mean that in nearly every case, if not all, a woman who wished an abortion could have one. A woman who is denied a desired lawful abortion and forced to continue an unwanted pregnancy would seem to face a greater risk of death, because of psychological factors, than the average woman, because the average includes all those women who wish to bear the child to term. The psychological factor alone, which under *Abarbanel* is a proper consideration, would seem to be decisive. Such a construction of the statute permitting voluntary abortions would render the statute virtually meaningless. Moreover, to determine the right to an abortion solely on the basis of the dangers of childbirth without regard to the relative dangers of the abortion would be contrary to good medical practice.

Nor can the statute be made certain by reading it as "substantially or reasonably" necessary to preserve the life of the mother. In the present context those terms are not sufficiently precise and would be subject to such different interpretations as to add little or nothing to "necessary." Thus, many people may feel that an abortion is reasonably or substantially necessary to preserve life where the risk of death is double or triple the ordinary risk in childbirth. Others may believe that anything which increases the possibility of death is a substantial risk which is not to be undertaken in the absence of countervailing considerations, so that "reasonably necessary" or "substantially necessary" becomes as destructive of the statute as "possibility of death." On the other hand, there may be those who feel that there is no reasonable or substantial necessity until it is more likely than not that the pregnant woman will not survive childbirth. Although in order contexts the implication of words such as "reasonably" and "substantially" may add certainty and avoid other due process objections, in the instant situation the implication of such words would merely increase the uncertainty.

There is one suggested test which is based on a policy underlying the statute and which would serve to make the statute certain. The test is probably in accord with the legislative intent at the time the statute was adopted. The Legislature may have intended in adopting the statute that abortion was permitted when the risk of death due to the abortion was less than the risk of death in childbirth and that otherwise abortion should be denied. As we have seen, at the time of the adoption of the statute abortion was a highly dangerous procedure, and under the relative safety test abortion would be permissible only where childbirth would be even more dangerous. In light of the test and the then existing medical practice, the question whether abortion should be limited to protect the embryo or fetus may have been immaterial because any such interest would be effectuated by limiting abortions to the rare cases where they were safer than childbirth.

The suggested test would involve an application of medical principles. Medical science may be able to tell us the proper method to treat a patient to minimize the risk of death, but without resort to matters outside medical competence, it cannot tell us the circumstances in which the safest treatment should be rejected and a more dangerous treatment followed in order to protect an embryo or fetus.

The new Therapeutic Abortion Act (Health & Saf. Code, §§ 25950-25954), has adopted a test analogous to the suggested one. Under the new statute, abortion is permissible during the first 20 weeks of pregnancy by a licensed physician in an accredited hospital (Health & Saf. Code, §§ 25951, 25953) if it is determined under prescribed procedures either that "There is substantial risk that continuance of the pregnancy would gravely impair the physical or mental health of the mother" (Health & Saf. Code, § 25951, subd. (c) 1), or that "The pregnancy resulted from rape or incest." (Health and Saf. Code, § 25951, subd. (c) 2.) Mental health includes mental illness to the extent that the woman would be dangerous to herself. (Health & Saf. Code, § 25954.) By limiting the abortion to the first 20 weeks, the Legislature has taken into account the danger to the mother of the later abortion and, by requiring the abortion to be performed by a licensed physician in an accredited hospital, has recognized the danger to the mother of other procedures. The further criteria for determining whether an abortion is permissible is the pregnant woman's physical and mental health. Thus, the test established is a medical one, whether the pregnant woman's physical and mental health will be furthered by abortion or by bearing the child to term, and the assessment does not involve considerations beyond medical competence. There is nothing to indicate that in adopting the Therapeutic Abortion Act the Legislature was asserting an interest in the embryo.

Although the suggested construction of former section 274, making abortion lawful where it is safer than childbirth and unlawful where abortion is more dangerous, may have been in accord with legislative intent, the statute may not be upheld against a claim of vagueness on the basis of such a construction. The language of the statute, "unless the same is necessary to preserve her life," does not suggest a relative safety test, and no case interpreting the statute has suggested that the statute be so construed. None of the parties or numerous amici who have filed briefs in the instant case suggest that the statute applies a relative safety test; to the contrary, the position of the parties and amici, including numerous lawyers, doctors, educators, clergymen and laymen, implies that the statute does not apply that standard. Thus, those claiming the statute is invalid urge that the only valid standard would be a relative safety test and that the statute fails to adopt such a test, and those urging the validity of the statute either state or imply that the standard applied is more restrictive. In the circumstances, we are satisfied that the statute may not be construed to adopt the relative safety test as against a claim of vagueness, because the language does not suggest that test and because of the practical evidence before us that men of "common" intelligence, indeed of uncommon intelligence, have not guessed at this meaning.*

*The practical aspects of the need to guess at the meaning of the abortion statute is shown by Packer & Gampell, Therapeutic Abortion: A Problem in Law and Medicine (1959) 11

5. The problem caused by the vagueness of the statute is accentuated because under the statute the doctor is, in effect, delegated the duty to determine whether a pregnant woman has the right to an abortion and the physician acts at his peril if he determines that the woman is entitled to an abortion. He is subject to prosecution for a felony and to deprivation of his right to practice medicine (Bus. & Prof.Code, § 2377) if his decision is wrong. Rather than being impartial, the physician has a "direct, personal, substantial, pecuniary interest in reaching a conclusion" that the woman should not have an abortion. The delegation of decision-making power to a directly involved individual violates the Fourteenth Amendment. *(Tumey v. Ohio* (1927) 273 U.S. 510, 523, 47 S.Ct. 437, 71 L.Ed. 749; see also *State Board of Dry Cleaners v. Thrift-D-Lux Cleaners,* 40 Cal.2d 436, 448, 254 P.2d 29 ["[T]he statute assumes to confer legislative authority upon those who are directly interested in the operation of the regulatory rule . . . ."]; *Blumenthal v. Board of Medical Examiners,* 57 Cal.2d 228, 235, 18 Cal.Rptr. 501, 504, 368 P.2d 101, 104.)

The inevitable effect of such delegation may be to deprive a woman of an abortion when under any definition of section 274 of the

Stan.L.Rev. 417. A questionnaire survey directed to 29 San Francisco Bay Area and Los Angeles hospitals *(id.,* at p. 423) based on hypothetical cases involving pregnant women seeking abortions yielded the following results *(id.,* at p. 444):

Case no.	Authors' evaluation of legality of abortion	Hospital would perform abortion Yes	No
1	Yes	21	1
2	No	10	12
3	No	6	16
4	No	15	7
5	No	8	13
6	No	8	14
7	Yes	17	4
8	No	5	17
9	Prob. Yes	10	11
10	Maybe	17	4
11	No	1	20

Penal Code, she would be entitled to such an operation, because the state, in delgating the power to decide when an abortion is necessary, has skewed the penalties in one direction; *no* criminal penalties are imposed where the doctor refuses to perform a necessary operation, even if the woman should in fact die because the operation was not performed.

The pressures on a physician to decide not to perform an absolutely necessary abortion are, under section 274 of the Penal Code, enormous, and because section 274 authorizes—and requires—the doctor to decide, at his peril, whether an abortion is necessary, a woman whose life is at stake may be as effectively condemned to death as if the law flatly prohibited all abortions.

To some extent the Therapeutic Abortion Act reduces these pressures. The act specifically authorizes an abortion by a licensed physician in an accredited hospital where the abortion is approved in advance by a committee of the medical staff of the hospital, applying medical standards. (Health & Saf.Code, § 25951.) At least in cases where there has been adherence to the procedural requirements of the statute, physicians may not be held criminally responsible, and a jury may not subsequently determine that the abortion was not authorized by statute.

6. We conclude that the validity of section 274 of the Penal Code before amendment cannot be sustained(14).

Since section 274 is invalid, Dr. Belous' conviction for violation of section 182 of the Penal Code, conspiracy to commit abortion, must likewise fall. The judgment is reversed with directions to the trial court to dismiss the indictment.

TRAYNOR, C. J., TOBRINER, J., and PIERCE,* J. pro tem., concur.

BURKE, Justice (dissenting). I dissent.

The defendant was found guilty by jury trial of a wilful violation of the abortion statute as it existed at the time of the offense. That he

*Assigned by the Chairman of the Judicial Council.

violated the statute is all but conceded in the briefs filed in his behalf.
Although he testified that he directed the young couple to a doctor,
unlicensed in California, because he believed that if they carried out
their threats of going to Tijuana to procure an abortion the young
woman's life would be in danger, he acknowledged upon cross-
examination that her life would not have been endangered if she were
not aborted. His assertions that he acted in good faith and out of
compassion are tainted somewhat by the evidence which showed that
he had referred other women to the same unlicensed physician on a
number of occasions and that he had participated on at least one-half of
those occasions in the fee paid the abortionist.

Had the doctor truly believed that the young woman's life was in
danger he could have done what was the common practice of taking the
patient to one of the several hospitals in which therapeutic abortions
were being performed. To my knowledge there is not one single instance
of a decision of the appellate courts of this state in which a doctor or a
hospital has been prosecuted for the performance of an abortion where
an independent hospital committee deemed the abortion to be
necessary to preserve the woman's life. The plain fact is, as the jury
found it to be, that this doctor, whatever his motive, possessed the
intent to assist in procuring the miscarriage of the woman for reasons
other than to preserve her life. This is the specific intent which the law
requires for conviction.

He supplied to the jury the answer an independent hospital
committee undoubtedly would have given him had he seen fit to seek its
approval for an abortion—the patient could bear the child without
endangering her life; therefore, to abort her would violate the law.

The threatened danger to the woman's life arose only from the
couple's assertions that they would seek an illegal abortion by an
unlicensed person. To assist them in attaining this goal was to flaunt his
profession's own standards and to aid in bringing about a direct
violation of the law.

The majority would reverse the conviction by declaring the
statute unconstitutional because of asserted uncertainty in the phrase,
"necessary to preserve [the woman's] life"(15). This phrase has been an
integral part of the California law against illegal abortions from the
time of its enactment in 1872 until the 1967 amendment to the section,
and similar language was in the original statute adopted in 1850(16).
Thus for over a hundred years in this state doctors, hospital committees,

judges, lawyers and juries have been called upon to give the phrase the common sense interpretation which the words appear to me to suggest. For this court over a hundred years later to find the language unconstitutionally vague and uncertain is a "negation of experience and common sense." *(United States v. Ragen,* 314 U.S. 513, 524, 62 S.Ct. 374, 379, 86 L.Ed. 383.)

Not only was the phrase long used in the California statute, it was also employed at common law (see, e.g., Perkins on Criminal Law (2d ed.) p. 145; Clark and Marshall, Crimes (6th ed.) pp. 688-689) and is or has been in the abortion statutes of many states (see e.g., Am.Jur. 2d, Abortion, § 9, p. 192; 153 A.L.R. 1218, 1266; Smith, Abortion and the Law (1967) p. 7). Implicit in the decisions of this court, as well as those of countless other courts, is the view that the phrase does not render such a statute invalid (see, e.g., *People v. Davis,* 43 Cal.2d 661, 276 P.2d 801; *People v. Gallardo,* 41 Cal.2d 57, 257 P.2d 29; *People v. Powell,* 34 Cal.2d 196, 208 P.2d 974; *People v. Wilson,* 25 Cal.2d 341, 153 P.2d 720; *People v. Rankin,* 10 Cal.2d 198, 74 P.2d 71). In *State v. Moretti,* 52 N.J. 182, 244 A.2d 499, 504 [cert. den. 393 U.S. 952, 89 S.Ct. 376, 21 L.Ed.2d 363] the court stated that when the phrase "lawful justification," as used in a statute prohibiting abortions done maliciously or without lawful justification, is confined "to the preservation of the mother's life," the statute is not subject to constitutional attack on the ground of vagueness. (See also *State v. Elliott,* 234 Or. 522, 383 P.2d 382, 384-385.)

The proper test as to certainty was stated by this court in *People v. Howard,* 70 A.C. 659, 665, 75 Cal.Rptr. 761, 764, 451 P.2d 401, 404, to be: "A statute should be sufficiently certain so that a person may know what is prohibited thereby and what may be done without violating its provisions, but it cannot be held void for uncertainty if any reasonable and practical construction can be given to its language. As stated in *Pacific Coast Dairy v. Police Court,* 214 Cal. 668, at page 676, 8 P.2d 140, 143, 80 A.L.R. 1217, 'Mere difficulty in ascertaining its meaning, or the fact that it is susceptible of different interpretations will not render it nugatory. Doubts as to its construction will not justify us in disregarding it.' [Citation.]"

The meaning of the phrase "necessary to preserve [the woman's] life" was considered in *People v. Ballard,* 167 Cal.App.2d 803, 814-815, 335 P.2d 204, 212, wherein the court stated, "Surely, the abortion statute (Pen.Code, § 274) does not mean by [this phrase] that the peril to life be imminent. It ought to be enough that the dangerous condition 'be potentially present, even though its full development might be delayed to a greater or less extent. Nor was it essential that the doctor should believe that the death of the patient would be otherwise *certain* in order to justify him in affording present relief.' *(State v. Dunklebarger,* 206 Iowa 971, 221 N.W. 592, 596; see also *Rex v. Bourne,* 1 K.B. 687 . . . ; *Commonwealth v. Wheeler,* 315 Mass. 394, 53 N.E.2d 4; 23 So. Cal.L.Rev. 523.) In *State v. Powers* . . . 155 Wash. 63, 67, 283 P. 439, 440, the court satisfied itself with an interpretation of 'necessity to save life' by stating, *'If the appellant in performing the operation did something which was recognized and approved by those reasonably skilled in his profession practicing in the same community . . . then it cannot be said that the operation was not necessary to preserve the life of the patient.'* " (Italics added.) (See also *People v. Abarbanel,* 239 Cal.App. 2d 31, 34, 48 Cal.Rptr. 336; *People v. Ballard,* 218 Cal.App.2d 295, 307, 32 Cal.Rptr. 233.)

Amici for appellant, 178 deans of medical schools, state that the italicized sentence quoted from *People v. Ballard, supra,* 167 Cal.App.2d 803, 814-815, 335 P.2d 204, is in error because "the medical profession has 'approved' abortions in cases [in which the objective was not to preserve the life of the woman and therefore] clearly outside of Penal Code section 274. Packer & Gampell, Therapeutic Abortion: A Problem in Law and Medicine, 11 Stan.L.Rev. 417, 447. . . . " However, that sentence must be understood to mean recognized and approved by such persons as being required to preserve the life of the patient.

The word "preserve" is defined in the dictionary as "1) To keep or save from injury or destruction; . . . to protect; save. 2) To keep in existence or intact; . . . To save from decomposition. . . . " (See Webster's New Internat. Dict. (3d ed. 1961).) As used in section 274, the word "preserve" has been regarded as synonymous with "save" (see, e.g., *People v. Kutz,* 187 Cal.App.2d 431, 436, 9 Cal.Rptr. 626; *People v. Malone,* 82 Cal.App.2d 54, 59, 185 P.2d 870; *Stern v. Superior Court,* 78 Cal.App.2d 9, 18, 177 P.2d 308), and to save a life ordinarily is understood as meaning to save from destruction, i.e. dying—not merely from injury. Thus the precipitation of a psychosis in the absence of a genuine threat of suicide is not a threat to life under section 274. (See Packer and Gampell, Therapeutic Abortion: A Problem in Law and Medicine, 11 Stan.L.Rev. 417, 433, 436.)

That the Legislature used the word "preserve" in the sense of save from destruction also appears from the purpose of the section. The law historically in various contexts has regarded the unborn child as a human being. (See Louisell, Abortion, The Practice of Medicine, and the Due Process of Law, 16 U.C.L.A. L.Rev. 233, 234-244.) Louisell (at p. 244) quotes from Prosser on Torts (3d ed. 1964) that "[M]edical authority has recognized long since that the child is in existence from the moment of conception, and for many purposes its existence is recognized by the law. The criminal law regards it as a separate entity, and the law of property considers it in being for all purposes which are to its benefit, such as taking by will or descent . . . All writers who have discussed the problem have joined . . . in maintaining that the unborn child in the path of an automobile is as much a person in the street as the mother." In *Raleigh Fitkin-Paul Morgan Mem. Hosp. v. Anderson*, 42 N.J. 421, 201 A.2d 537, 538 [cert. den. 377 U.S. 985, 84 S.Ct. 1894, 12 L.Ed.2d 1032] it was held that an unborn child of a woman who did not wish blood transfusions because they were contrary to her religious convictions was entitled to the law's protection and that an order would be made to insure such transfusions to the mother in the event they are necessary in the opinion of the attending physician.

Several statutes show that the California law has been in accord in regarding the unborn child as a human being for various purposes. (See, e.g., Pen.Code, §§ 3706 and 270; Civ.Code, § 29)(17). In *Scott v. McPheeters*, 33 Cal.App.2d 629, 634, 92 P.2d 678, 681, the court declared: "The respondent asserts that the provisions of section 29 of the Civil Code are based on a fiction of law to the effect that an unborn child is a human being separate and distinct from its mother. We think that assumption of our statute is not a fiction, but upon the contrary that it is an established and recognized fact by science and by everyone of understanding."

It is reasonable to believe that section 274, as it read at the time in question, was not an exception to the law's attitude respecting the unborn child as a human being and that it was designed to protect no only the mother's life but also that of the child. In view of that purpose it would appear that the Legislature intended that the child would be deprived of his right to life only if in the absence of an abortion there was a danger of the mother's death—not merely of injury to her.

" '[T]he Constitution does not require impossible standards'; all that is required is that the language 'conveys sufficiently definite warning as to the proscribed conduct when measured by common understanding and practices . . . .' *United States v. Petrillo*, 332 U.S. 1,

7-8, 67 S.Ct. 1538, 91 L.Ed. 1877." *(Roth v. United States,* 354 U.S. 476, 491, 77 S.Ct. 1304, 1312, 1 L.Ed.2d 1498.) The phrase in question, when applied according to the standard heretofore stated (namely, whether persons reasonably skilled in their profession practicing in the same community recognized and approved the act as being required to save the patient from dying) clearly gives such warning.

Furthermore, section 274 punishes only those who act with " '. . . the intent to commit a criminal abortion, that is, an abortion for a purpose other than to preserve [i.e. save from destruction] the life of the mother.' " *(People v. Abarbanel, supra,* 239 Cal.App.2d 31, 34-35, 48 Cal.Rptr. 336, 339; *People v. Ballard, supra,* 167 Cal.App.2d 803, 817, 335 P.2d 204.) The requirement of such an intent eviscerates much of the majority's claim that the section is impermissibly vague. (See generally *Mishkin v. New York,* 383 U.S. 502, 507, fn. 5, 86 S.Ct. 958, 16 L.Ed.2d 56; *Boyce Motor Lines, Inc. v. United States,* 342 U.S. 337, 342, 72 S.Ct. 329, 96 L.Ed. 367.) A person who performs an abortion with such an intent has fair warning that his conduct may violate the law even though he may not be certain where the jury will draw the line on the matter of necessity.

The principal cases relied upon by the majority, in which statutes have been declared unconstitutionally vague, do not support such a finding when applied to the abortion statute. In *People v. McCaughan,* 49 Cal.2d 409, 317 P.2d 974, the statute prohibited, among other conduct, "harsh" or "unkind" treatment of a mentally ill person. These words were held not to have an established meaning either at common law or as a result of adjudication. They were held unconstitutionally vague. On the other hand, the phrase "neglect of duty" and the word "cruel" were upheld because they did have such well established meanings, just as do the words utilized in the phrase under attack here.

Lanzetta v. New Jersey, 306 U.S. 451, 453, 59 S.Ct. 618, 83 L.Ed. 888, construed a statute defining "gangster" and making it a crime for anyone to be such a person. The phrase "consisting of two or more persons" was all that purported to define "gang," and the word "gang" was held so vague and uncertain as to violate the Fourteenth Amendment.

Connally v. General Const. Co., 269 U.S. 385, 395, 46 S.Ct. 126, 128, 129, 70 L.Ed. 322, involved a statute requiring a contractor to pay his employees "not less than the *current rate of . . . wages* in the *locality* where the work is performed," and the court held the italicized words unconstitutionally vague. Unlike the statute involved here, the statute in question was a new statute and the court noted that its application "depends, not upon a word of fixed meaning in itself, or one made definite by statutory or judicial definition. . . . "

In contrast to these cases, here the challenged statute has a fixed meaning, frequently applied and impliedly interpreted by the courts in the more than one hundred years of its existence. In addition, the statute requires proof of the specific intent to commit a criminal abortion before a person may be successfully prosecuted under it.

There is, of course, a presumption in favor of constitutionality, and the invalidity of a legislative act must be clear before it can be declared unconstitutional. (In re Anderson, 69 Cal.2d 613, 628, 73 Cal.Rptr. 21, 447 P.2d 117.)

The majority cite no authority holding that the term "necessary to preserve [the woman's] life" is impermissibly vague, and I agree with the conclusion as to the constitutionality of the section that is implicit in the multitude of past decisions affirming convictions for illegal abortion, and for murder where death was the result of such an act.

I would affirm the judgment.

McCOMB and SULLIVAN, JJ., concur.

SULLIVAN, Justice (dissenting).

I concur in the views of Justice BURKE. Reading the majority's attack on Penal Code section 274, one would think that the English language which has been the sensitive instrument of our system of law for over 500 years, has lost, by the mere passage of time, all capacity for clarity of expression. The majority strike down the statute solely because they find so vague and uncertain as to offend constitutional standards of due process, a single brief clause of nine words of long and common usage: "unless the same is necessary to preserve her life." There is no mystique enveloping the statute and, as Justice BURKE points out, the clause now challenged has stood the test of over a hundred years, and presumably of countless human incidents falling within its scope, apparently without evoking a single whimpering cry against it.

The mandate of the section is plain and clear, and simply means this: no one shall intentionally procure the miscarriage of a woman unless it is necessary to save her life. "The criminal intent necessary to support a conviction of illegal abortion must show that it was performed for a purpose other than to save [the abortee's] life." *(People v. Abarbanel* (1965) 239 Cal.App.2d 31, 34, 48 Cal.Rptr. 336, 338.) I dare say that the average man in the street, confronted with this law, would have little trouble in extracting its sense (we hold him accountable to much more complicated enactments); and the doctor, with his professional training and expertise would have even less. We have said that "[i]t is a cardinal rule, to be applied to the interpretation of particular words, phrases, or clauses in a statute or a Constitution, that the entire substance of the instrument or of that portion thereof which has relation to the subject under review should be looked to in order to determine the scope and purpose of the particular provision therein of which such words, phrases, or clauses form a part, and in order also to determine the particular intent of the framers of the instrument in that portion thereof wherein such words, phrases, or clauses appear." *(Wallace v. Payne* (1925) 197 Cal. 539, 544, 241 P.879, 881). In the case before us, the challenged clause when so examined, is clear in meaning.

Yet the majority, by engaging in a process of elaborate and lavish analysis, transform that which is simple and lucid into something complex and arcane. Actually the analysis is focused on only three words: "necessary to preserve." Their fair equivalent is "necessary to save" (see *People v. Abarbanel, supra,* 239 Cal.App.2d 31, 34, 48 Cal.Rptr. 336; *People v. Ballard* (1959) 167 Cal.App.2d 803, 814, 817, 335 P.2d 204). Rather than evaluate these words in the light of "the entire substance" (see *Wallace v. Payne, supra,* 197 Cal. 539, 544, 241 P.879), the majority resort to a dissection: "There is, of course, no standard definition of 'necessary to preserve,' and taking the words separately, no clear meaning emerges." (Majority opn., p. 358.) In support of this thesis, it is asserted that the word "necessary" does not have a "fixed meaning." In general, few words do(18). It is further insisted that the definition of "preserve" is "even less enlightening." Accordingly, the majority discard its obvious meaning, that is, "save," as used in the context "to save a life." From such analysis, the opinion concludes "that the term 'necessary to preserve' in section 274 of the Penal Code is not susceptible of a construction that does not violate legislative intent and that is sufficiently certain to satisfy due process requirements without improperly infringing on fundamental constitutional rights." (Majority opn., p. 357) Actually the gist of this is that the three words "necessary to preserve" are so shrouded in darkness that the average man cannot detect what they mean although average men and men above average have had no trouble with them for a hundred years.

I cannot accept so tortured a conclusion, wrenched from a statute which has had its roots in the law's historic solicitude for the priceless gift of life. The statute plainly prohibits an abortion unless it is necessary to save the mother's life. It strains reason to say that this crystal-clear exception to the law is "so vague that men of common intelligence must necessarily guess at its meaning . . . ." *(Lanzetta v. New Jersey* (1939) 306 U.S. 451, 453, 59 S.Ct. 618, 619, 83 L.Ed. 888—see majority opn., p. 357.) And it strains credulity to assume that this defendant, who under the evidence wilfully violated the statute, had to engage in any such guesswork with respect to the law governing his conduct.

I would affirm the judgment.

McCOMB, J., concurs.

Rehearing denied; McCOMB, BURKE and SULLIVAN, JJ., dissenting.

PIERCE, J., sitting pro tem. in place of MOSK, J., who deemed himself disqualified.

REFERENCES

1. Stats.1850, ch. 99, § 45, at p. 233: "[E]very person who shall administer or cause to be administered or taken, any medicinal substances, or shall use or cause to be used any instruments whatever, with the intention to procure the miscarriage of any woman then being with child, and shall be thereof duly convicted, shall be punished by imprisonment in the State Prison for a term not less than two years, nor more than five years: *Provided,* that no physician shall be affected by the last clause of this section, who, in the discharge of his professional duties, deems it necessary to produce the miscarriage of any woman in order to save her life."

2. Penal Code, section 274, as amended reads: "Every person who provides, supplies, or administers to any woman, or procures any woman to take any medicine, drug, or substance, or uses or employs any instrument or other means whatever, with intent thereby to procure the miscarriage of such woman, . . . *except as provided in the Therapeutic Abortion Act . . . of the Health and Safety Code,* is punishable by imprisonment in the state prison . . . ." (Stats.1967, ch. 327, § 3, at p. 1523; italics added.)

    The Therapeutic Abortion Act (Health & Saf. Code, §§ 25950-25954) authorizes abortions "only" if the abortion takes place in an accredited hospital (§ 25951, subd. (a)); the abortion is approved by a hospital staff committee consisting of at least three licensed physicians and surgeons (§ 25951, subd. (b)); and there is "substantial risk that continuance of the pregnancy would gravely impair the physical or mental health of the mother" (§ 25951, subd. (c) (1)); the pregnancy resulted from rape or incest (§ 25951, subd. (c) (2)); or the woman is under 15 years of age (§ 25952, subd. (c)).

3. Compare United States v. Harriss (1954) 347 U.S. 612, 634, 74 S.Ct. 808, 820, 98 L.Ed. 989 (dissenting opinion): "Whoever kidnaps, steals, kills, or commits similar acts of violence upon another is bound to know that he is inviting retribution by society, and many of the statutes which define these long-established crimes are traditionally and perhaps necessarily vague."

4. The definitions suggested by the two *Ballard* cases and by *Abarbanel* will be discussed later in this opinion.

5. Dr. Belous' standing to raise this right is unchallenged. (Cf. Griswold v. Connecticut (1965) 381 U.S. 479, 481, 85 S.Ct. 1678, 14 L.Ed.2d 510; Barrows v. Jackson (1953) 346 U.S. 249, 257, 73 S.Ct. 1031, 97 L.Ed. 1586; Parrish v. Civil Service Commission, 66 Cal.2d 260, 264, 57 Cal.Rptr. 623, 425 P.2d 223.)

6. E.g., The maternal death rate in 1966 was 0.5 per 100,000 population and 29.1 per 100,000 births. (Statistical Abstract of the United States (1968) table 73, at p. 58, table 68, at p. 55.) In California in 1966 the maternal death rate was 2.1 per 10,000 live births. (California Statistical Abstract (1968) table E-3, at p. 67.) As to a particular pregnant woman the risk of death may be greater or lesser.

7.   C. Tietze & H. Lehfeldt, Legal Abortion in Eastern Europe (April
      1961) 175 J.A.M.A. 1149, 1152; see also V. Kolblova, Legal
      Abortion in Czechoslovakia (April 1966) 196 J.A.M.A. 371; K.-H.
      Mehland, Combatting Illegal Abortion in the Socialist Countries
      of Europe (1966) 13 World Med.J. 84. There are, of course, no
      comparable data in the United States. However, in California
      from November 1967 through September 1968, 3,775 therapeutic
      abortions were reported without a maternal death. (See Annual
      Report on the Implementation of the Therapeutic Abortion Act,
      Department of Public Health, Bureau of Maternal and Child
      Health (January 1969), table 1.)
      The only data contrary to the conclusions above is provided by
      amicus for respondent, relying on Swedish data showing that
      maternal mortality from abortion is slightly higher than maternal
      mortality from giving birth. The Swedish figures are, however,
      explainable by the fact that abortions in Sweden are often
      performed during late pregnancy. (See Tietze & Lehfeldt, *supra*,
      175 J.A.M.A. 1149, 1152 (e.g., in 1949, 35 percent of Swedish
      abortions were performed after the first trimester); Hoffmeyer,
      Medical Aspects of the Danish Legislation on Abortions (1965) 17
      W.Res.L.Rev. 529, 544-545.)
8.   The phrases "criminal abortion" and "illegal abortion" are used
      by the medical profession—and by legal commentators—to
      encompass all abortions obtained other than from a physician in
      an accepted surgical environment. Any use of the phrase "criminal
      abortion" or "illegal abortion" in this opinion merely adopts the
      common phraseology; no legal conclusion is intended.
9.   There is considerable literature describing the experience of
      various hospitals with infected abortion. Hospital experience,
      however, can be assumed to be only the tip of the iceberg. Many
      badly infected women will be treated at home or in a doctor's
      office. (Reid, Assessment and Management of the Seriously Ill
      Patient Following Abortion (March 1967) 199 J.A.M.A. p. 805.)
      See, for hospital data, Goodno, Cushner, Molumphey, Manage-
      ment of Infected Abortion (1963) 85 Am.J.Obst. & Gynec. 16
      [Baltimore City Hospitals]; Knapp, Platt and Douglas, Septic
      Abortion (1960) 15 Obst. & Gynec. 344 [The New York Hospital];
      Moritz & Thompson, Septic Abortion (1966) 95 Am.J.Obst. &
      Gynec. 46 [Miami Valley Hospital, Dayton, Ohio]; Stevenson &

Yang, Septic Abortion With Shock (1962) 83 Am.J.Obst. & Gynec. 1229 [Detroit Receiving Hospital]; Studdiford & Douglas, Placental Bacteremia: A Significant Finding in Septic Abortion Accompanied by Vascular Collapse (1956) 71 Am.J.Obst. & Gynec. 842 [Bellevue Hospital, New York].)

10. One of the amici in support of respondent agrees: "There is a substantial risk that abortions performed by persons in unregulated places, will bring injury or even death to the mother." Authorities recognizing and discussing the tragic health problem created by illegal abortions are legion. (See, e.g., Bates, The Abortion Mill: An Institutional Study (1954) 45 J.Crim.L.C. & P.S. 157; Eastman, Expectant Motherhood (3d ed. 1957) 106 et seq.; Gold, Erhardt, Jacobziner & Nelson, Therapeutic Abortions in New York City: A 20-Year Review (1965) 55 Am.J.Pub.Health 964, 970-971; Guttmacher (ed. 1967) The Case for Legalized Abortion Now; Lader (1966) Abortion; Leavy & Kummer, Criminal Abortion; Human Hardship and Unyielding Laws (1962) 35 So.Cal.L.Rev. 123; Lucas, Federal Constitutional Limitations on the Enforcement and Administration of State Abortion Statutes (1968) 46 N.C.L.Rev. 730; Niswander, Medical Abortion Practices in the United States (1965) 17 W.Res.L.Rev. 403.)

11. It has been pointed out that "embryo" is more accurately descriptive than "fetus" in the instant case. Webster's New International Dictionary, *supra*, states: " . . . In mammals . . . *embryo* is applied only to early stages passed within the mother's body; later (in human embryology, usually after the third month of development) the young is called a *fetus*. . . . " (Italics in original.)

12. Statutes classifying the unborn child as the same as the born child require that the child be born alive for the provisions to apply. (E.g., Civ.Code, § 29 ["A child conceived, but not yet born, is to be deemed an existing person, so far as may be necessary for its interests in the event of its subsequent birth; . . . "]; Prob.Code, § 250 ["A posthumous child is considered as living at the death of the parent."]; Prob.Code, § 255 [An illegitimate child is the heir of his mother, "whether born or conceived."].) Similarly, cases holding that a child can recover for injuries caused before his birth require that the child be born alive. The

interest protected is that of the child; and the right attaches, not to the embryo or fetus, but to the living child. (Scott v. McPheeters, 33 Cal.App.2d 629, 637, 92 P.2d 678, 93 P.2d 562 [child injured at birth can bring action for injuries]; see also, Carroll v. Skloff (1964), 415 Pa. 47, 202 A.2d 9, 11; Tomlin v. Laws (1922) 301 Ill. 616, 134 N.E. 24, 25; Prosser, Law of Torts (3d ed.1964) at p. 356 ["The child, provided that he is born alive, is permitted to maintain an action . . . "].)

Where the embryo or fetus is allowed to assert rights before birth it is the prospective mother or parents who are bringing the action; thus it is their interest that the law protects. (Kyne v. Kyne, 38 Cal.App.2d 122, 127-128, 100 P.2d 806 [action on behalf of unborn child for support and to establish paternity]; People v. Sianes, 134 Cal.App. 355, 357-358, 25 P.2d 487 [criminal action for nonsupport against father of unborn child]; People v. Yates, 114 Cal.App.Supp. 782, 786, 298 P. 961 [same].) Similarly, in those jurisdictions which recognize a cause of action for the loss of an unborn child, it is the parents' "distressing wrong in the loss of a child" that the law has recognized. (Prosser, *supra*, § 56, at p. 357; Torigian v. Watertown News Co. Inc. (1967) 352 Mass. 446, 448, 225 N.E.2d 926.)

In a case involving a pregnant woman who refused a blood transfusion, in ordering the transfusion the court made clear that it was concerned with the woman, rather than the fetus: " . . . Mrs. Jones wanted to live." (Application of President & Directors of Georgetown Col. (1964) 118 U.S.App.D.C. 90, 331 F.2d 1000, 1009, cert. denied, 377 U.S. 978, 84 S.Ct. 1883, 12 L.Ed.2d 746, but see Raleigh Fitkin-Paul Morgan Mem. Hosp. v. Anderson (1964) 42 N.J. 421, 201 A.2d 537, 538, cert. denied, 377 U.S. 985, 84 S.Ct. 1894, 12 L.Ed.2d 1032, suggesting that an 8-month pregnant woman could be required to have blood transfusions to protect the unborn child.)

Although sections 3705 and 3706 of the Penal Code, which provide for suspending the execution of a pregnant woman, reflect an interest in the unborn child, the sections do not affect any other significant private interests and thus furnish no basis to evaluate the interest protected or to conclude that the embryo or fetus is equivalent to a born child.

13. One case has held that, for purposes of the manslaughter and murder statutes, human life may exist where childbirth has commenced but has not been fully completed. (People v. Chavez 77 Cal.App.2d 621, 624, 626, 176 P.2d 92.)

14. It has been urged that the Therapeutic Abortion Act is unconstitutional because it contains uncertainties similar to those in the repealed statute, because it infringes on the woman's right to choose whether to bear children, and because the act does not expressly permit an abortion where there is a likelihood that a deformed child will be born. Since the act was adopted after the abortion in the instant case, we do not reach the issue of its validity.

15. Section 274 then read: "Every person who provides, supplies, or administers to any woman, or procures any woman to take any medicine, drug, or substance, or uses or employs any instrument or other means whatever, with intent thereby to procure the miscarriage of such woman, unless the same is *necessary to preserve her life,* is punishable . . . " (Italics added.)

16. The 1850 statute (ch. 99, § 45, p. 233) provided that every person who did any of the enumerated acts with a specified intent shall be punishable *"Provided,* that no physician shall be affected . . . who, in the discharge of his professional duties, deems it necessary to produce the miscarriage of any woman in order to save her life."

17. Penal Code section 3706 requires that the execution of a death penalty be suspended if the defendant is pregnant and without regard to the stage of pregnancy.

   Penal Code section 270 makes punishable a father's wilful failure to provide a minor child with necessary items and provides that "A child conceived but not yet born is to be deemed an existing person in so far as this section is concerned."

   Civil Code section 29 provides in part that "A child conceived, but not yet born, is to be deemed an existing person, so far as may be necessary for its interests in the event of its subsequent birth . . . "

18. "Words, however, do not have absolute and constant referents. 'A word is a symbol of thought but has no arbitrary and fixed meaning like a symbol of algebra or chemistry, . . . ' (Pearson v. State Social Welfare Board (1960) 54 Cal.2d 184, 195, 5 Cal.Rptr.

553, 559, 353 P.2d 33, 39.) The meaning of particular words or groups of words varies with the ' . . . verbal context and surrounding circumstances and purposes in view of the linguistic education and experience of their users and their hearers or readers (not excluding judges). . . . A word has not meaning apart from these factors; much less does it have an objective meaning, one true meaning.' (Corbin, The Interpretation of Words and the Parole Evidence Rule (1965) 50 Cornell L.Q. 161, 187.)" (Pacific Gas & E. Co. v. G. W. Thomas Drayage Etc. Co. (1968) 69 Cal.2d 33, 38, 69 Cal.Rptr. 561, 564, 442 P.2d 641, 644.)

"Words are used in an endless variety of contexts. Their meaning is not subsequently attached to them by the reader but is formulated by the writer and can only be found by interpretation in the light of all the circumstances that reveal the sense in which the writer used the words." (Universal Sales Corp. v. Cal. etc. Mfg. Co. (1942) 20 Cal.2d 751, 776, 128 P.2d 665, 679, Traynor, J. concurring.)

INDEX